2. Scrambled Eggs:
Eggs, milk, butter, cheese, spinach.

Ingredient:

• 6 eggs
• 2 tablespoons milk
• 1 tablespoon butter
• 1 cup fresh spinach, chopped
• 1/4 cup shredded cheddar or Swiss cheese

Instructions:

1. In a medium bowl, whisk together the eggs and milk until well combined.

2. Melt the butter in a nonstick skillet over medium heat.

3. Add the egg mixture to the skillet and let it sit for 20•30 seconds to set the bottom slightly.

4. Using a spatula, gently push the eggs from the side of the pan into the center, tilting the pan to allow the uncooked egg to flow to the edges.

5. When the eggs are still slightly wet, add the chopped spinach and shredded cheese.

6. Continue stirring and folding the eggs gently until they reach your desired doneness, about 2•3 minutes total.

7. Season with salt and pepper to taste.

8. Serve the scrambled eggs immediately while hot.

Enjoy your cheesy, veggie•packed scrambled eggs!

3. Oatmeal with Fruit:
Oats, milk, honey, blueberries, bananas.

Ingredient:

• 1 cup old•fashioned rolled oats
• 1 1/2 cups milk (dairy, almond, or oat milk)
• 1 tablespoon honey (or maple syrup)
• 1/2 cup fresh or frozen blueberries
• 1 ripe banana, sliced

Instructions:

1. In a medium saucepan, combine the oats and milk. Bring to a simmer over medium heat, stirring occasionally.

2. Once the oats have thickened to your desired consistency, about 5•7 minutes, remove from heat.

3. Stir in the honey until well combined.

4. Top the oatmeal with the fresh or frozen blueberries and sliced banana.

5. Serve the oatmeal warm, garnished with any additional toppings you'd like, such as:
• Chopped nuts or seeds
• Shredded coconut
• Cinnamon

Enjoy your nutritious and delicious oatmeal breakfast! The combination of creamy oats, sweet fruit, and a touch of honey makes for a satisfying and wholesome meal.

Welcome to ***"5-Ingredient Cookbook for College Students: Fast, Fresh, and Budget-Friendly Recipes for Students"!*** College life is a whirlwind of classes, study sessions, social events, and maybe even a part-time job. With such a hectic schedule, it can be challenging to find time to cook, let alone whip up something healthy and delicious. That's where this cookbook comes in.

This book is designed with you, the busy college student, in mind. Here, you'll find over 115 recipes that require just five simple ingredients. These meals are quick to prepare, easy on your wallet, and packed with fresh flavors. Whether you're a seasoned cook or a kitchen novice, these recipes will help you create tasty dishes without the hassle of complicated cooking techniques or long ingredient lists.

Why Five Ingredients?

Using only five ingredients keeps things simple and manageable. It means fewer trips to the grocery store, less time spent prepping, and more time to enjoy your meal and get back to your studies (or your Netflix binge). But simplicity doesn't mean sacrificing taste. Each recipe is carefully crafted to ensure that every ingredient plays a crucial role in delivering maximum flavor.

What You'll Find Inside

In this cookbook, you'll discover a variety of recipes that cover every meal of the day:

- ***Breakfast Boosters:*** Start your day right with quick and nutritious breakfast options.

- ***Hearty Lunches:*** Power through your day with satisfying and easy-to-make lunches.

- ***Simple Suppers:*** End your day with delicious dinners that are ready in a flash.

- ***Snacks and Sides:*** Find the perfect accompaniments for your meals or something to munch on during study breaks.

- ***Sweet Treats***: Indulge your sweet tooth with simple desserts that don't require a ton of ingredients.

So grab your apron, gather your ingredients, and get ready to embark on a culinary adventure. With this book as your guide, you'll be whipping up fast, fresh, and budget-friendly meals in no time. Happy cooking!

1. Avocado Toast: Bread, avocado, lemon juice, red pepper flakes, cherry tomatoes.

Ingredient:

1. Bread (your choice of bread)
2. Avocado, mashed
3. Lemon juice
4. Red pepper flakes
5. Cherry tomatoes, halved

Instructions:

1. Toast the bread to your desired level of crispness.

2. Spread the mashed avocado evenly over the toasted bread.

3. Drizzle a bit of lemon juice over the avocado.

4. Sprinkle red pepper flakes over the top.

5. Top with halved cherry tomatoes.

That's it! This easy 5•ingredient recipe makes a delicious and nutritious avocado toast. The combination of the creamy avocado, tangy lemon, and the kick of the red pepper flakes creates a flavorful and satisfying snack or light meal.

4. Smoothie Bowl:
Frozen berries, banana, yogurt, granola, chia seeds.

Ingredient:

- 1 cup frozen mixed berries (such as blueberries, raspberries, strawberries)
- 1 ripe banana
- 1 cup plain Greek yogurt
- 2 tablespoons granola
- 1 tablespoon chia seeds

Instructions:

1. In a blender, combine the frozen berries, banana, and yogurt. Blend until smooth and creamy.

2. Pour the smoothie into a bowl.

3. Top the smoothie with the granola and chia seeds.

Optional Toppings:
- Sliced fresh fruit (such as banana, kiwi, or mango)
- Toasted coconut flakes
- Chopped nuts or seeds
- A drizzle of honey or maple syrup

Enjoy your nutrient•dense smoothie bowl! The combination of the creamy smoothie base, crunchy granola, and fresh toppings makes for a satisfying and wholesome breakfast or snack.

5. Pancakes:
Flour, milk, eggs, sugar, baking powder.

Ingredient:

- 1 cup all•purpose flour
- 2 teaspoons baking powder
- 1 tablespoon sugar
- 1/4 teaspoon salt
- 1 cup milk
- 1 egg
- 2 tablespoons melted butter or oil

Instructions:

1. In a medium bowl, whisk together the flour, baking powder, sugar, and salt.

2. In a separate bowl, whisk together the milk, egg, and melted butter or oil.

3. Pour the milk mixture into the flour mixture and whisk just until combined (do not overmix).

4. Heat a lightly oiled griddle or nonstick skillet over medium heat.

5. For each pancake, pour about 1/4 cup of the batter onto the griddle. Cook until bubbles appear on the surface, about 2•3 minutes.

6. Flip the pancakes and cook until golden brown on the other side, about 1•2 minutes more.

7. Serve the pancakes warm, with your desired toppings such as:
- Maple syrup
- Fresh fruit (berries, bananas, etc.)
- Whipped cream
- Chocolate chips or nuts

Enjoy your homemade fluffy pancakes! This basic recipe can be easily customized with different mix•ins or toppings.

6. Breakfast Burrito:
Tortilla, eggs, cheese, black beans, salsa.

Ingredient:

- 1 large flour tortilla
- 2 eggs, scrambled
- 1/4 cup shredded cheddar or Monterey Jack cheese
- 1/3 cup black beans, drained and rinsed
- 2 tablespoons salsa

Instructions:

1. Warm the tortilla according to package instructions, or in a dry skillet over medium heat for 30 seconds per side.

2. In a small bowl, scramble the eggs.

3. Place the warm tortilla on a plate. Layer the scrambled eggs, shredded cheese, black beans, and salsa down the center of the tortilla.

4. Fold the bottom of the tortilla up over the filling, then fold in the sides and continue rolling up tightly into a burrito shape.

5. Serve the breakfast burrito immediately.

That's it! Just 5 simple ingredients • tortilla, eggs, cheese, black beans, and salsa • for a satisfying and portable breakfast burrito. Adjust the fillings to your taste preferences.

7. Greek Yogurt Parfait:
Greek yogurt, honey, granola, strawberries, almonds.

Ingredient:

- 1 cup plain Greek yogurt
- 2 tablespoons honey
- 1/2 cup granola
- 1 cup fresh strawberries, sliced
- 2 tablespoons sliced almonds

Instructions:

1. In a parfait glass or bowl, layer half of the Greek yogurt.

2. Drizzle 1 tablespoon of the honey over the yogurt.

3. Sprinkle half of the granola over the honey.

4. Layer half of the sliced strawberries over the granola.

5. Repeat the layers, starting with the remaining yogurt, then honey, granola, and strawberries.

6. Top the parfait with the sliced almonds.

7. Serve chilled or at room temperature.

That's it! Just 5 simple ingredients • Greek yogurt, honey, granola, strawberries, and almonds • for a delicious and nutritious parfait. You can easily adjust the amounts of each ingredient to suit your taste preferences.

8. French Toast:
Bread, eggs, milk, cinnamon, maple syrup.

Ingredient:

• 4 slices of bread (such as challah, brioche, or sourdough)
• 2 eggs
• 1/2 cup milk
• 1 teaspoon ground cinnamon
• 2 tablespoons maple syrup (plus more for serving)

Instructions:

1. In a shallow bowl, whisk together the eggs, milk, and cinnamon until well combined.

2. Dip each slice of bread into the egg mixture, coating both sides evenly.

3. Heat a lightly oiled griddle or nonstick skillet over medium heat.

4. Cook the French toast slices for 2•3 minutes per side, or until golden brown.

5. Serve the French toast warm, drizzled with additional maple syrup.

Optional Toppings:
• Powdered sugar
• Fresh berries
• Whipped cream
• Chopped nuts

That's it! Just 5 simple ingredients • bread, eggs, milk, cinnamon, and maple syrup • for a delicious and classic French toast. Adjust the amounts as needed to make more or less servings. Enjoy your homemade French toast!

9. Bagel with Cream Cheese:
Bagel, cream cheese, smoked salmon, capers, red onion.

Ingredient:
- 1 bagel, toasted
- 2 tablespoons cream cheese
- 2 ounces smoked salmon
- 1 tablespoon capers, drained
- 2 tablespoons thinly sliced red onion

Instructions:

1. Toast the bagel until lightly golden brown.

2. Spread the cream cheese evenly over the toasted bagel.

3. Top the cream cheese with the smoked salmon, capers, and sliced red onion.

4. Serve immediately.

Optional Additions:
- Chopped fresh dill
- Sliced cucumber
- Cracked black pepper

That's it! Just 5 simple ingredients • a bagel, cream cheese, smoked salmon, capers, and red onion • for a delicious and satisfying breakfast or brunch. The combination of the savory salmon, tangy capers, and crisp onion pairs perfectly with the creamy cream cheese on the toasted bagel. Adjust the amounts of each ingredient to your taste preferences.

10. Egg Muffins:
Eggs, spinach, cherry tomatoes, cheese, bell pepper.

Ingredient:

• 6 eggs
• 1 cup chopped fresh spinach
• 1/2 cup halved cherry tomatoes
• 1/4 cup shredded cheddar or feta cheese
• 1/4 cup diced bell pepper (any color)
• Salt and pepper to taste

Instructions:

1. Preheat your oven to 350°F (175°C). Grease a 6•cup muffin tin.

2. In a medium bowl, whisk the eggs together.

3. Stir in the chopped spinach, halved cherry tomatoes, shredded cheese, and diced bell pepper. Season with salt and pepper.

4. Divide the egg mixture evenly among the 6 muffin cups.

5. Bake for 18•20 minutes, or until the eggs are set and the muffins are lightly golden.

6. Allow the egg muffins to cool for 5 minutes before removing them from the tin.

Serve the egg muffins warm. They make a great portable breakfast or snack.

That's it! Just 5 main ingredients • eggs, spinach, cherry tomatoes, cheese, and bell pepper • for these delicious and nutritious egg muffins. Feel free to customize the fillings to your liking.

11. Breakfast Sandwich:
English muffin, egg, cheese, ham, avocado.

Ingredient:

- 1 English muffin, split in half
- 1 egg
- 1 slice cheddar or Swiss cheese
- 1 slice ham
- 1/4 avocado, sliced

Instructions:

1. Toast the English muffin halves until lightly golden.

2. In a small nonstick skillet, cook the egg over medium heat until the whites are set and the yolk is cooked to your desired doneness, about 2•3 minutes.

3. Place the cooked egg on the bottom half of the toasted English muffin.

4. Top the egg with the slice of cheese.

5. Add the slice of ham on top of the cheese.

6. Arrange the avocado slices on top of the ham.

7. Place the top half of the English muffin on the sandwich.

8. Serve the breakfast sandwich immediately while warm.

That's it! Just 5 simple ingredients • English muffin, egg, cheese, ham, and avocado • for a satisfying and delicious breakfast sandwich. You can customize the fillings to your liking, such as using a different type of cheese or adding other toppings like tomato or spinach.

12. Chia Pudding:
Chia seeds, almond milk, honey, vanilla extract, berries.

Ingredient:

• 1/4 cup chia seeds
• 1 cup unsweetened almond milk
• 1 tablespoon honey
• 1 teaspoon vanilla extract
• 1/2 cup mixed berries (such as blueberries, raspberries, strawberries)

Instructions:

1. In a medium bowl, whisk together the chia seeds, almond milk, honey, and vanilla extract until well combined.

2. Cover the bowl and refrigerate for at least 2 hours, or up to 24 hours, stirring occasionally, until the chia seeds have thickened the mixture into a pudding•like consistency.

3. When ready to serve, divide the chia pudding into 2 serving bowls or glasses.

4. Top each portion with 1/4 cup of the mixed berries.

Optional Toppings:
• Chopped nuts or seeds
• Shredded coconut
• Cinnamon

That's it! Just 5 simple ingredients • chia seeds, almond milk, honey, vanilla, and berries • for a nutritious and delicious chia pudding. The chia seeds provide fiber, protein, and omega•3s, while the berries add natural sweetness and antioxidants. Adjust the amounts of each ingredient to suit your taste preferences.

13. Breakfast Quesadilla:
Tortilla, eggs, cheese, black beans, salsa.

Ingredient:

- 2 medium flour tortillas
- 2 eggs, scrambled
- 1/4 cup shredded cheddar or Monterey Jack cheese
- 1/3 cup black beans, drained and rinsed
- 2 tablespoons salsa

Instructions:

1. In a nonstick skillet over medium heat, scramble the eggs until cooked through. Transfer the eggs to a plate.

2. Place one tortilla in the skillet and top with half of the scrambled eggs, black beans, shredded cheese, and salsa.

3. Top with the second tortilla.

4. Cook the quesadilla for 2•3 minutes per side, or until the tortilla is lightly golden and the cheese is melted.

5. Remove the quesadilla from the skillet and slice into wedges.

6. Repeat the process with the remaining ingredients to make a second quesadilla.

Serve the breakfast quesadillas warm, with extra salsa on the side if desired.

That's it! Just 5 simple ingredients • tortilla, eggs, cheese, black beans, and salsa • for a satisfying and portable breakfast quesadilla. You can customize the fillings to your liking.

14. Mango Smoothie:
Mango, banana, yogurt, honey, ice.

Ingredient:
- 1 cup frozen mango chunks
- 1 ripe banana
- 1 cup plain Greek yogurt
- 1 tablespoon honey
- 1/2 cup ice cubes

Instructions:

1. In a blender, combine the frozen mango chunks, banana, Greek yogurt, honey, and ice cubes.

2. Blend on high speed until the mixture is smooth and creamy, about 1•2 minutes.

3. Pour the mango smoothie into a glass.

Optional Variations:
- Add a splash of milk or plant•based milk for a thinner consistency.
- Substitute the honey with maple syrup or agave nectar.
- Add a handful of spinach or kale for extra nutrients.
- Top with sliced fresh mango, toasted coconut, or a sprinkle of cinnamon.

That's it! Just 5 simple ingredients • mango, banana, yogurt, honey, and ice • for a delicious and refreshing mango smoothie. The combination of sweet mango, creamy yogurt, and a touch of honey makes for a perfectly balanced and satisfying smoothie. Adjust the amounts of each ingredient to suit your taste preferences.

15. Granola Bars:
Oats, peanut butter, honey, chocolate chips, nuts.

Ingredient:

- 2 cups old·fashioned rolled oats
- 1/2 cup creamy peanut butter
- 1/3 cup honey
- 1/3 cup chocolate chips
- 1/4 cup chopped nuts (such as almonds, walnuts, or pecans)

Instructions:

1. Line an 8x8 inch baking pan with parchment paper, leaving some overhang on the sides for easy removal.

2. In a large bowl, mix together the rolled oats, peanut butter, and honey until well combined.

3. Fold in the chocolate chips and chopped nuts.

4. Press the mixture firmly into the prepared baking pan, using your hands or the back of a spoon to compact it.

5. Refrigerate the granola bars for at least 2 hours, or until firm.

6. Lift the granola bars out of the pan using the parchment paper overhang. Cut into 8·10 bars.

Store the granola bars in an airtight container in the refrigerator for up to 1 week.

That's it! Just 5 simple ingredients · oats, peanut butter, honey, chocolate chips, and nuts · for these homemade granola bars. You can customize the mix·ins to your liking, such as using different types of nuts or dried fruit.

16. Chicken Caesar Wrap: Tortilla, chicken breast, romaine lettuce, Caesar dressing, Parmesan cheese.

Ingredient:

- 1 large flour tortilla
- 4 oz grilled or roasted chicken breast, sliced or shredded
- 1 cup chopped romaine lettuce
- 2 tablespoons Caesar dressing
- 2 tablespoons grated Parmesan cheese

Instructions:

1. Lay the tortilla flat on a clean surface.

2. Layer the sliced or shredded chicken breast down the center of the tortilla.

3. Top the chicken with the chopped romaine lettuce.

4. Drizzle the Caesar dressing over the lettuce.

5. Sprinkle the grated Parmesan cheese over the top.

6. Fold the bottom of the tortilla up over the filling, then fold in the sides and continue rolling up tightly into a wrap.

7. Slice the wrap in half diagonally, if desired, and serve immediately.

That's it! Just 5 simple ingredients • tortilla, chicken, romaine, Caesar dressing, and Parmesan • for a delicious and portable Chicken Caesar Wrap. You can use grilled, roasted, or even leftover chicken for this recipe. Adjust the amounts of each ingredient to your taste preferences.

17. Caprese Sandwich:
Bread, mozzarella, tomato, basil, balsamic glaze.

Ingredient:

• 2 slices of bread (such as sourdough or ciabatta)
• 2•3 slices of fresh mozzarella cheese
• 1•2 slices of ripe tomato
• 3•4 fresh basil leaves
• 1•2 tablespoons balsamic glaze

Instructions:

1. Place one slice of bread on a clean surface.

2. Layer the mozzarella cheese slices on top of the bread.

3. Add the tomato slices in an even layer.

4. Tear or chiffonade the fresh basil leaves and sprinkle them over the tomatoes.

5. Drizzle the balsamic glaze over the basil and tomatoes.

6. Top with the second slice of bread to complete the sandwich.

7. Slice the sandwich in half diagonally, if desired.

That's it! Just 5 simple ingredients • bread, mozzarella, tomato, basil, and balsamic glaze • for a delicious and fresh Caprese Sandwich. You can use any type of bread you prefer, and adjust the amounts of each ingredient to your taste. The combination of creamy mozzarella, juicy tomatoes, fragrant basil, and tangy balsamic glaze makes for a flavorful and satisfying sandwich.

18. Hummus and Veggie Wrap:
Tortilla, hummus, cucumber, bell pepper, spinach.

Ingredient:
- 1 large whole wheat or spinach tortilla
- 2•3 tablespoons hummus
- 1/4 cup sliced cucumber
- 1/4 cup sliced bell pepper (any color)
- 1/2 cup fresh spinach leaves

Instructions:

1. Lay the tortilla flat on a clean surface.

2. Spread the hummus evenly over the center of the tortilla.

3. Layer the sliced cucumber and bell pepper over the hummus.

4. Top with the fresh spinach leaves.

5. Fold the bottom of the tortilla up over the filling, then fold in the sides and continue rolling up tightly into a wrap.

6. Slice the wrap in half diagonally, if desired.

That's it! Just 5 simple ingredients • tortilla, hummus, cucumber, bell pepper, and spinach • for a nutritious and flavorful Hummus and Veggie Wrap. You can use any type of tortilla or wrap you prefer, and adjust the amounts of the vegetables to your liking. The creamy hummus pairs perfectly with the fresh, crunchy veggies for a satisfying and portable meal or snack.

19. Grilled Cheese Sandwich:
Bread, cheddar cheese, butter, tomato, bacon.

Ingredient:

- 2 slices of bread (such as sourdough or white)
- 2•3 slices of cheddar cheese
- 1 tablespoon butter, softened
- 1 slice of tomato
- 2 slices of cooked bacon

Instructions:

1. Butter one side of each slice of bread.

2. Place one slice of bread, butter•side down, in a skillet or griddle over medium heat.

3. Layer the cheddar cheese slices on top of the bread.

4. Top the cheese with the tomato slice and bacon slices.

5. Place the second slice of bread, butter•side up, on top of the sandwich.

6. Cook the sandwich for 2•3 minutes per side, or until the bread is golden brown and the cheese is melted.

7. Remove the grilled cheese sandwich from the heat and let it cool for a minute before serving.

That's it! Just 5 simple ingredients • bread, cheddar cheese, butter, tomato, and bacon • for a delicious and classic grilled cheese sandwich. You can customize the fillings to your liking, such as using different types of cheese or adding other toppings like avocado or caramelized onions.

20. Chicken Salad:
Chicken breast, mayonnaise, celery, grapes, almonds.

Ingredient:

- 2 cups cooked and shredded or diced chicken breast
- 1/2 cup mayonnaise
- 1/2 cup diced celery
- 1/2 cup halved grapes
- 1/4 cup chopped toasted almonds

Instructions:

1. In a medium bowl, combine the shredded or diced chicken, mayonnaise, diced celery, halved grapes, and chopped almonds.

2. Stir the ingredients together until the chicken salad is well mixed and coated in the mayonnaise.

3. Taste and adjust any seasonings as needed, such as adding a pinch of salt and pepper.

4. Serve the chicken salad on bread, crackers, or lettuce leaves.

That's it! Just 5 simple ingredients • chicken, mayonnaise, celery, grapes, and almonds • for a delicious and versatile chicken salad. You can use rotisserie chicken or leftover cooked chicken to make this recipe even easier. Adjust the amounts of each ingredient to your taste preferences.

21. Tuna Salad:
Canned tuna, mayonnaise, celery, onion, pickle relish.

Ingredient:

• 2 (5 oz) cans of tuna, drained
• 1/4 cup mayonnaise
• 1/4 cup diced celery
• 2 tablespoons finely chopped onion
• 2 tablespoons pickle relish

Instructions:

1. In a medium bowl, combine the drained tuna, mayonnaise, diced celery, chopped onion, and pickle relish.

2. Stir the ingredients together until the tuna salad is well mixed and coated in the mayonnaise.

3. Taste and adjust any seasonings as needed, such as adding a pinch of salt and pepper.

4. Serve the tuna salad on bread, crackers, or lettuce leaves.

Optional Additions:
• Hard boiled egg, chopped
• Diced dill pickle
• Chopped fresh parsley or dill
• Squeeze of lemon juice

That's it! Just 5 simple ingredients • tuna, mayonnaise, celery, onion, and pickle relish • for a classic and flavorful tuna salad. You can customize the ingredients to your taste preferences. Enjoy this tuna salad as a sandwich, on top of greens, or with crackers.

22. BLT Sandwich:
Bread, bacon, lettuce, tomato, mayonnaise.

Ingredient:

• 2 slices of bread (such as sourdough or whole wheat)
• 3•4 slices of cooked bacon
• 2•3 leaves of lettuce, washed and patted dry
• 1•2 slices of tomato
• 2 tablespoons mayonnaise

Instructions:

1. Toast the bread slices until lightly golden brown.

2. Spread the mayonnaise evenly on one slice of the toasted bread.

3. Layer the cooked bacon slices on top of the mayonnaise.

4. Add the lettuce leaves, overlapping them slightly.

5. Top with the tomato slices.

6. Place the second slice of toasted bread on top to complete the sandwich.

7. Cut the BLT in half diagonally, if desired.

That's it! Just 5 simple ingredients • bread, bacon, lettuce, tomato, and mayonnaise • for a classic and delicious BLT sandwich. You can use your choice of bread, adjust the amounts of each ingredient, and add any other toppings you enjoy, such as avocado or a sprinkle of black pepper.

23. Quinoa Salad:
Quinoa, cucumber, cherry tomatoes, feta cheese, lemon juice.

Ingredient:

- 1 cup cooked quinoa, cooled
- 1/2 cup diced cucumber
- 1/2 cup halved cherry tomatoes
- 1/4 cup crumbled feta cheese
- 2 tablespoons fresh lemon juice

Instructions:

1. In a medium bowl, combine the cooked and cooled quinoa, diced cucumber, halved cherry tomatoes, and crumbled feta cheese.

2. Drizzle the fresh lemon juice over the salad and gently toss to coat the ingredients.

3. Taste and adjust any seasonings as needed, such as adding a pinch of salt and pepper.

4. Serve the quinoa salad chilled or at room temperature.

Optional Additions:
- Chopped fresh herbs (parsley, mint, basil)
- Toasted nuts or seeds
- Diced red onion
- Kalamata olives

That's it! Just 5 simple ingredients • quinoa, cucumber, cherry tomatoes, feta cheese, and lemon juice • for a refreshing and flavorful quinoa salad. The combination of the nutty quinoa, crisp veggies, tangy feta, and bright lemon makes for a delicious and nutritious side dish or light meal. Adjust the amounts of each ingredient to your taste preferences.

24. Greek Salad:
Cucumber, tomatoes, red onion, olives, feta cheese.

Ingredient:

- 1 cucumber, diced
- 2•3 tomatoes, diced
- 1/2 red onion, thinly sliced
- 1/2 cup pitted kalamata olives, halved
- 4 oz feta cheese, crumbled
- 2 tbsp olive oil
- 1 tbsp red wine vinegar
- 1 tsp dried oregano
- Salt and pepper to taste

Instructions:

1. In a large bowl, combine the diced cucumber, tomatoes, sliced red onion, and halved olives.

2. Crumble the feta cheese over the top.

3. In a small bowl, whisk together the olive oil, red wine vinegar, and dried oregano. Season with salt and pepper.

4. Drizzle the dressing over the salad and gently toss to coat.

5. Let the salad sit for 5•10 minutes to allow the flavors to meld together.

6. Serve chilled or at room temperature.

Enjoy your fresh and flavorful Greek salad! Let me know if you need any clarification on the recipe.

25. Pasta Salad:
Pasta, cherry tomatoes, mozzarella, basil, balsamic vinegar.

Ingredient:

- 8 oz pasta (such as fusilli or penne), cooked and cooled
- 1 pint cherry tomatoes, halved
- 8 oz fresh mozzarella cheese, cubed
- 1/4 cup fresh basil leaves, chopped
- 2 tbsp balsamic vinegar

Instructions:

1. Cook the pasta according to package instructions. Drain and rinse with cold water to cool completely.

2. In a large bowl, combine the cooked and cooled pasta, halved cherry tomatoes, cubed mozzarella, and chopped fresh basil.

3. Drizzle the balsamic vinegar over the salad and gently toss to coat everything evenly.

4. Refrigerate the pasta salad for at least 30 minutes to allow the flavors to meld.

5. Serve chilled or at room temperature.

That's it! Just 5 simple ingredients • pasta, tomatoes, mozzarella, basil, and balsamic vinegar • for a delicious and refreshing pasta salad. Let me know if you need any clarification on the recipe.

26. Turkey and Cheese Sandwich:
Bread, turkey, cheese, lettuce, mustard.

Ingredient:
- 2 slices of bread (your choice of bread)
- 2•3 slices of turkey
- 1•2 slices of cheese (such as cheddar or Swiss)
- 1•2 leaves of lettuce
- 1•2 tsp of mustard

Instructions:

1. Lay the two slices of bread on a clean surface.

2. Spread the mustard evenly on one slice of bread.

3. Layer the turkey slices on top of the mustard.

4. Place the cheese slices on top of the turkey.

5. Top the cheese with the lettuce leaves.

6. Place the other slice of bread on top to complete the sandwich.

That's it! Just 5 simple ingredients • bread, turkey, cheese, lettuce, and mustard • for a delicious and satisfying turkey and cheese sandwich. You can adjust the amounts of each ingredient to your personal preference.

27. Egg Salad:
Eggs, mayonnaise, mustard, celery, green onion.

Ingredient:

- 6 hard•boiled eggs, peeled and chopped
- 1/4 cup mayonnaise
- 1 tsp Dijon mustard
- 1/4 cup diced celery
- 2 tbsp sliced green onions

Instructions:

1. In a medium bowl, combine the chopped hard•boiled eggs.

2. Add the mayonnaise and Dijon mustard. Stir to coat the eggs evenly.

3. Fold in the diced celery and sliced green onions.

4. Season with salt and pepper to taste.

5. Chill the egg salad in the refrigerator for at least 30 minutes before serving to allow the flavors to meld.

That's it! Just 5 simple ingredients • eggs, mayonnaise, mustard, celery, and green onions • for a delicious and creamy egg salad. You can adjust the amounts of each ingredient to your personal preference.

28. Veggie Stir•Fry:
Broccoli, bell pepper, soy sauce, garlic, tofu.

Ingredient:

• 1 head of broccoli, cut into florets
• 1 bell pepper, sliced
• 2 cloves of garlic, minced
• 1/4 cup soy sauce
• 1 block of firm tofu, cubed

Instructions:

1. Heat a large skillet or wok over medium•high heat. Add a tablespoon of oil.

2. Add the broccoli florets and sliced bell pepper to the hot pan. Stir•fry for 3•4 minutes until the vegetables start to soften.

3. Add the minced garlic and stir•fry for an additional minute until fragrant.

4. Pour in the soy sauce and gently toss the vegetables to coat them evenly.

5. Add the cubed tofu and continue to stir•fry for 2•3 minutes, until the tofu is heated through and the vegetables are tender•crisp.

6. Serve the veggie stir•fry immediately, over rice or noodles if desired.

That's it! Just 5 simple ingredients • broccoli, bell pepper, garlic, soy sauce, and tofu • for a delicious and nutritious veggie stir•fry. You can adjust the amounts of each ingredient to your personal preference.

29. Chicken and Rice:
Chicken breast, rice, broccoli, soy sauce, garlic.

Ingredient:

- 1 lb boneless, skinless chicken breasts, cubed
- 1 cup uncooked white rice
- 2 cups broccoli florets
- 2 cloves garlic, minced
- 2 tbsp soy sauce

Instructions:

1. In a medium saucepan, cook the rice according to package instructions.

2. While the rice is cooking, heat a large skillet or wok over medium•high heat. Add a tablespoon of oil.

3. Add the cubed chicken to the hot pan and cook for 5•7 minutes, until the chicken is cooked through and no longer pink.

4. Add the broccoli florets and minced garlic to the pan. Stir•fry for 3•4 minutes until the broccoli is tender•crisp.

5. Pour in the soy sauce and stir to coat the chicken and broccoli evenly.

6. Once the rice is cooked, fluff it with a fork and add it to the skillet. Gently toss everything together until well combined.

7. Serve the chicken and rice immediately.

That's it! Just 5 simple ingredients • chicken, rice, broccoli, garlic, and soy sauce • for a delicious and easy one•pan meal. You can adjust the amounts of each ingredient to your personal preference.

30. Taco Salad:
Ground beef, lettuce, cheese, salsa, tortilla chips.

Ingredient:

- 1 lb ground beef
- 1 head of lettuce, chopped
- 1 cup shredded cheese (cheddar or Mexican blend)
- 1 cup salsa
- 2 cups tortilla chips, crushed

Instructions:

1. In a large skillet, cook the ground beef over medium•high heat until browned and crumbled, about 5•7 minutes. Drain any excess fat.

2. In a large salad bowl, combine the chopped lettuce, cooked ground beef, shredded cheese, and salsa. Toss gently to mix.

3. Top the taco salad with the crushed tortilla chips.

4. Serve the taco salad immediately, or refrigerate until ready to serve.

That's it! Just 5 simple ingredients • ground beef, lettuce, cheese, salsa, and tortilla chips • for a delicious and easy taco salad. You can adjust the amounts of each ingredient to your personal preference.

31. Spaghetti Aglio e Olio:
Spaghetti, garlic, olive oil, red pepper flakes, parsley.

Ingredient:

- 8 oz spaghetti
- 4 cloves garlic, thinly sliced
- 1/4 cup olive oil
- 1/4 tsp red pepper flakes
- 2 tbsp chopped fresh parsley

Instructions:

1. Bring a large pot of salted water to a boil. Cook the spaghetti according to package instructions until al dente. Drain and set aside.

2. In a large skillet, heat the olive oil over medium heat. Add the sliced garlic and cook for 1•2 minutes, stirring frequently, until fragrant and just starting to turn golden.

3. Reduce the heat to low and add the red pepper flakes. Cook for 30 seconds, stirring constantly, to infuse the oil with the pepper flavor.

4. Add the cooked spaghetti to the skillet and toss to coat the noodles evenly with the garlic•infused oil.

5. Remove from heat and stir in the chopped fresh parsley. Season with salt and pepper to taste.

6. Serve the Spaghetti Aglio e Olio immediately, while hot.

That's it! Just 5 simple ingredients • spaghetti, garlic, olive oil, red pepper flakes, and parsley • for this classic Italian pasta dish. Adjust the amounts of each ingredient to your personal taste preferences.

32. Chicken Alfredo: Chicken breast, fettuccine, Alfredo sauce, Parmesan cheese, broccoli.

Ingredient:

- 1 lb boneless, skinless chicken breasts, cubed
- 8 oz fettuccine pasta
- 1 jar (15 oz) Alfredo sauce
- 1/2 cup grated Parmesan cheese
- 2 cups broccoli florets

Instructions:

1. Bring a large pot of salted water to a boil. Cook the fettuccine according to package instructions until al dente. Drain and set aside.

2. In a large skillet, cook the cubed chicken over medium•high heat until no longer pink, about 6•8 minutes. Remove the chicken from the skillet and set aside.

3. In the same skillet, add the broccoli florets and a splash of water. Cover and steam the broccoli for 3•4 minutes until tender•crisp.

4. Reduce the heat to low and add the Alfredo sauce to the skillet with the broccoli. Stir to combine.

5. Add the cooked fettuccine and the cooked chicken to the skillet. Toss everything together until the pasta is evenly coated with the Alfredo sauce.

6. Sprinkle the grated Parmesan cheese over the top and serve immediately.

That's it! Just 5 simple ingredients • chicken, fettuccine, Alfredo sauce, Parmesan cheese, and broccoli • for a delicious and creamy Chicken Alfredo dish. Adjust the amounts of each ingredient to your personal taste preferences.

33. Tacos:
Tortillas, ground beef, cheese, lettuce, salsa.

Ingredient:

- 8•10 small corn or flour tortillas
- 1 lb ground beef
- 1 cup shredded cheese (cheddar or Mexican blend)
- 1 cup shredded lettuce
- 1 cup salsa

Instructions:

1. In a large skillet, cook the ground beef over medium•high heat until browned and crumbled, about 5•7 minutes. Drain any excess fat.

2. Warm the tortillas according to package instructions, either in a dry skillet or wrapped in a damp paper towel and microwaved for 30 seconds.

3. To assemble the tacos, place a spoonful of the cooked ground beef in the center of each tortilla.

4. Top the beef with shredded cheese, shredded lettuce, and a spoonful of salsa.

5. Serve the tacos immediately, with any additional toppings or condiments on the side.

That's it! Just 5 simple ingredients • tortillas, ground beef, cheese, lettuce, and salsa • for delicious and customizable tacos. You can adjust the amounts of each ingredient to your personal preference.

34. Baked Ziti: Ziti pasta, marinara sauce, ricotta cheese, mozzarella, Italian sausage.

Ingredient:

- 12 oz ziti pasta
- 1 jar (24 oz) marinara sauce
- 1 cup ricotta cheese
- 2 cups shredded mozzarella cheese
- 1 lb Italian sausage, cooked and crumbled

Instructions:

1. Preheat your oven to 375°F.

2. Cook the ziti pasta according to package instructions until al dente. Drain and set aside.

3. In a large bowl, combine the cooked ziti, marinara sauce, ricotta cheese, and crumbled Italian sausage. Mix well.

4. Transfer the ziti mixture to a 9x13 inch baking dish. Spread it out evenly.

5. Sprinkle the shredded mozzarella cheese over the top.

6. Bake for 20•25 minutes, or until the cheese is melted and bubbly.

7. Let the baked ziti cool for 5 minutes before serving.

That's it! Just 5 simple ingredients • ziti pasta, marinara sauce, ricotta cheese, mozzarella cheese, and Italian sausage • for a delicious and comforting baked ziti dish. You can adjust the amounts of each ingredient to your personal preference.

35. Stuffed Bell Peppers:
Bell peppers, ground beef, rice, tomato sauce, cheese.

Ingredient:

• 4 bell peppers, halved and seeded
• 1 lb ground beef
• 1 cup cooked rice
• 1 (15 oz) can tomato sauce
• 1 cup shredded cheese (cheddar or mozzarella)

Instructions:

1. Preheat your oven to 375°F.

2. In a large skillet, cook the ground beef over medium heat until browned and crumbled, about 5•7 minutes. Drain any excess fat.

3. In a bowl, mix the cooked ground beef, cooked rice, and 1/2 cup of the tomato sauce until well combined.

4. Arrange the bell pepper halves in a baking dish. Spoon the beef and rice mixture evenly into the pepper halves.

5. Pour the remaining tomato sauce over the stuffed peppers.

6. Sprinkle the shredded cheese over the top.

7. Bake for 25•30 minutes, or until the peppers are tender and the cheese is melted and bubbly.

8. Serve the stuffed bell peppers hot.

That's it! Just 5 simple ingredients • bell peppers, ground beef, rice, tomato sauce, and cheese • for a delicious and easy stuffed bell pepper dish. You can adjust the amounts of each ingredient to your personal preference.

36. Chicken Stir•Fry:
Chicken breast, bell pepper, broccoli, soy sauce, garlic.

Ingredient:

- 1 lb boneless, skinless chicken breasts, cut into bite•sized pieces
- 1 bell pepper, sliced
- 2 cups broccoli florets
- 2 cloves garlic, minced
- 2 tbsp soy sauce

Instructions:

1. In a large skillet or wok, heat a tablespoon of oil over medium•high heat.

2. Add the cubed chicken to the hot pan and cook for 5•7 minutes, until the chicken is cooked through and no longer pink.

3. Add the sliced bell pepper and broccoli florets to the pan. Stir•fry for 3•4 minutes, until the vegetables are tender•crisp.

4. Stir in the minced garlic and soy sauce. Toss everything together to coat the chicken and vegetables evenly.

5. Continue to stir•fry for an additional 1•2 minutes, until the garlic is fragrant.

6. Serve the chicken stir•fry immediately, over rice or noodles if desired.

That's it! Just 5 simple ingredients • chicken, bell pepper, broccoli, garlic, and soy sauce • for a delicious and easy chicken stir•fry. You can adjust the amounts of each ingredient to your personal preference.

37. BBQ Chicken Pizza:
Pizza dough, BBQ sauce, chicken breast, red onion, cheese.

Ingredient:

- 1 lb pizza dough
- 1/2 cup BBQ sauce
- 1 lb boneless, skinless chicken breasts, cooked and shredded
- 1/2 red onion, thinly sliced
- 1 1/2 cups shredded cheese (mozzarella or cheddar)

Instructions:

1. Preheat your oven to 450°F. If using a pizza stone, place it in the oven to preheat as well.

2. Roll or stretch the pizza dough out into a 12•inch circle on a lightly floured surface.

3. Spread the BBQ sauce evenly over the pizza dough, leaving a 1/2•inch border.

4. Sprinkle the shredded chicken evenly over the BBQ sauce.

5. Top with the sliced red onion and shredded cheese.

6. Transfer the pizza to the preheated pizza stone or baking sheet.

7. Bake for 12•15 minutes, or until the crust is golden brown and the cheese is melted and bubbly.

8. Slice and serve the BBQ Chicken Pizza immediately.

That's it! Just 5 simple ingredients • pizza dough, BBQ sauce, chicken, red onion, and cheese • for a delicious and easy BBQ Chicken Pizza. You can adjust the amounts of each ingredient to your personal preference.

38. Salmon and Asparagus:
Salmon fillet, asparagus, lemon, garlic, dill.

Ingredient:

• 4 salmon fillets (about 1 lb total)
• 1 lb asparagus, trimmed
• 1 lemon, cut into wedges
• 2 cloves garlic, minced
• 2 tbsp chopped fresh dill

Instructions:

1. Preheat your oven to 400°F.

2. Arrange the salmon fillets and asparagus spears on a large baking sheet.

3. Drizzle the salmon and asparagus with a little olive oil and season with salt and pepper.

4. Sprinkle the minced garlic and chopped dill over the top.

5. Bake for 12•15 minutes, or until the salmon is cooked through and the asparagus is tender.

6. Serve the salmon and asparagus immediately, with the lemon wedges on the side.

That's it! Just 5 simple ingredients • salmon, asparagus, lemon, garlic, and dill • for a delicious and healthy salmon and vegetable dish. You can adjust the amounts of each ingredient to your personal preference.

39. Fajitas: Chicken breast, bell peppers, onion, tortillas, fajita seasoning.

Ingredient:

- 1 lb boneless, skinless chicken breasts, sliced into strips
- 2 bell peppers, sliced into strips
- 1 onion, sliced into strips
- 8•10 small flour or corn tortillas
- 2 tbsp fajita seasoning

Instructions:

1. In a large skillet or wok, heat a tablespoon of oil over medium•high heat.

2. Add the sliced chicken to the hot pan and cook for 5•7 minutes, until the chicken is cooked through and no longer pink.

3. Add the sliced bell peppers and onion to the pan. Sprinkle the fajita seasoning over the chicken and vegetables.

4. Stir•fry the chicken and vegetables for 5•7 minutes, until the peppers and onions are tender•crisp.

5. Warm the tortillas according to package instructions, either in a dry skillet or wrapped in a damp paper towel and microwaved for 30 seconds.

6. To serve, place some of the chicken and vegetable mixture into the center of each warm tortilla.

That's it! Just 5 simple ingredients • chicken, bell peppers, onion, tortillas, and fajita seasoning • for delicious and easy chicken fajitas. You can adjust the amounts of each ingredient to your personal preference.

40. Chili: Ground beef, kidney beans, diced tomatoes, chili powder, onion.

Ingredient:

- 1 lb ground beef
- 1 (15 oz) can kidney beans, drained and rinsed
- 1 (14.5 oz) can diced tomatoes
- 2 tbsp chili powder
- 1 onion, diced

Instructions:

1. In a large pot or Dutch oven, cook the ground beef over medium•high heat until browned and crumbled, about 5•7 minutes. Drain any excess fat.

2. Add the diced onion to the pot and cook for 2•3 minutes, until the onion is translucent.

3. Stir in the chili powder and cook for 1 minute to toast the spices.

4. Add the drained and rinsed kidney beans and the can of diced tomatoes (with their juices) to the pot.

5. Bring the chili to a simmer and let it cook for 15•20 minutes, stirring occasionally, to allow the flavors to meld.

6. Taste and adjust seasoning as needed, adding more chili powder for a spicier chili.

7. Serve the chili hot, with desired toppings such as shredded cheese, sour cream, or chopped green onions.

That's it! Just 5 simple ingredients • ground beef, kidney beans, diced tomatoes, chili powder, and onion • for a delicious and easy homemade chili. You can adjust the amounts of each ingredient to your personal preference.

41. Baked Chicken:
Chicken thighs, garlic, rosemary, lemon, potatoes.

Ingredient:

- 8 bone•in, skin•on chicken thighs
- 4 cloves garlic, minced
- 2 tbsp chopped fresh rosemary
- 1 lemon, cut into wedges
- 1 lb baby potatoes, halved

Instructions:

1. Preheat your oven to 400°F.

2. Arrange the chicken thighs and halved potatoes in a large baking dish or on a rimmed baking sheet.

3. Sprinkle the minced garlic and chopped rosemary evenly over the chicken and potatoes.

4. Squeeze the juice from the lemon wedges over the chicken and potatoes, then place the lemon wedges around the dish.

5. Season the chicken and potatoes with salt and pepper.

6. Bake for 40•45 minutes, or until the chicken is cooked through and the potatoes are tender.

7. Broil for 2•3 minutes at the end to crisp up the chicken skin, if desired.

8. Serve the baked chicken and potatoes immediately, with the roasted lemon wedges.

That's it! Just 5 simple ingredients • chicken thighs, garlic, rosemary, lemon, and potatoes • for a delicious and easy baked chicken dish. You can adjust the amounts of each ingredient to your personal preference.

42. Lemon Butter Shrimp:
Shrimp, butter, garlic, lemon, parsley.

Ingredient:
- 1 lb large shrimp, peeled and deveined
- 4 tbsp unsalted butter
- 3 cloves garlic, minced
- 1 lemon, juiced and zested
- 2 tbsp chopped fresh parsley

Instructions:

1. In a large skillet, melt the butter over medium heat.

2. Add the minced garlic and cook for 1 minute, until fragrant.

3. Add the shrimp to the skillet and cook for 2·3 minutes per side, until the shrimp are pink and opaque.

4. Squeeze the lemon juice over the shrimp and sprinkle the lemon zest on top.

5. Remove the skillet from heat and stir in the chopped fresh parsley.

6. Serve the lemon butter shrimp immediately, with the sauce spooned over the top.

That's it! Just 5 simple ingredients • shrimp, butter, garlic, lemon, and parsley • for a delicious and easy lemon butter shrimp dish. You can adjust the amounts of each ingredient to your personal preference.

43. Mac and Cheese:
Pasta, cheddar cheese, milk, butter, flour.

Ingredient:

- 8 oz elbow macaroni
- 2 cups shredded cheddar cheese
- 1 cup milk
- 2 tbsp unsalted butter
- 2 tbsp all•purpose flour

Instructions:

1. Cook the elbow macaroni according to package instructions. Drain and set aside.

2. In a medium saucepan, melt the butter over medium heat. Whisk in the flour and cook for 1 minute.

3. Gradually whisk in the milk and bring the mixture to a simmer. Cook, stirring frequently, until the sauce thickens, about 3•5 minutes.

4. Remove the saucepan from heat and stir in the shredded cheddar cheese until it's melted and the sauce is smooth.

5. Add the cooked macaroni to the cheese sauce and stir to combine.

6. Serve the mac and cheese hot.

That's it! Just 5 simple ingredients • pasta, cheddar cheese, milk, butter, and flour • for a creamy and delicious mac and cheese. You can adjust the amounts of each ingredient to your personal preference.

44. Meatloaf:
Ground beef, breadcrumbs, egg, ketchup, onion.

Ingredient:

- 1 lb ground beef
- 1 cup breadcrumbs
- 1 egg, beaten
- 1/2 cup ketchup
- 1 onion, finely chopped

Instructions:

1. Preheat your oven to 375°F.

2. In a large bowl, combine the ground beef, breadcrumbs, beaten egg, ketchup, and chopped onion. Mix well until all the ingredients are evenly incorporated.

3. Transfer the meatloaf mixture to a loaf pan or shape it into a loaf on a baking sheet.

4. Bake for 50•60 minutes, or until the internal temperature reaches 160°F.

5. Let the meatloaf rest for 5•10 minutes before slicing and serving.

That's it! Just 5 simple ingredients • ground beef, breadcrumbs, egg, ketchup, and onion • for a classic and delicious meatloaf. You can adjust the amounts of each ingredient to your personal preference.

Some optional additions could include:
- 1 tbsp Worcestershire sauce
- 1 tsp dried oregano or basil
- 1/4 cup grated Parmesan cheese

45. Curry Chicken:
Chicken breast, curry powder, coconut milk, onion, spinach.

Ingredient:

- 1 lb boneless, skinless chicken breasts, cubed
- 2 tbsp curry powder
- 1 (13.5 oz) can coconut milk
- 1 onion, diced
- 2 cups fresh spinach leaves

Instructions:

1. In a large skillet or wok, heat a tablespoon of oil over medium•high heat.

2. Add the cubed chicken to the hot pan and cook for 5•7 minutes, until the chicken is cooked through and no longer pink.

3. Add the diced onion to the pan and cook for 2•3 minutes, until the onion is translucent.

4. Sprinkle the curry powder over the chicken and onion, and stir to coat everything evenly.

5. Pour in the can of coconut milk and stir to combine. Bring the mixture to a simmer.

6. Add the fresh spinach leaves to the pan and cook for 2•3 minutes, until the spinach is wilted.

7. Serve the curry chicken immediately, over rice if desired.

That's it! Just 5 simple ingredients • chicken, curry powder, coconut milk, onion, and spinach • for a flavorful and easy curry chicken dish. You can adjust the amounts of each ingredient to your personal preference.

46. Shepherd's Pie:
Ground beef, mashed potatoes, carrots, peas, onion.

Ingredient:

• 1 lb ground beef
• 1 onion, diced
• 2 cups frozen peas and carrots
• 3 cups mashed potatoes (homemade or store•bought)
• Salt and pepper to taste

Instructions:

1. Preheat your oven to 375°F.

2. In a large skillet, cook the ground beef over medium•high heat until browned and crumbled, about 5•7 minutes. Drain any excess fat.

3. Add the diced onion to the skillet and cook for 2•3 minutes, until the onion is translucent.

4. Stir in the frozen peas and carrots and cook for an additional 2•3 minutes.

5. Season the beef mixture with salt and pepper to taste.

6. Spread the beef and vegetable mixture in the bottom of a 9x13 inch baking dish.

7. Spread the mashed potatoes evenly over the top of the beef mixture.

8. Bake for 25•30 minutes, or until the potatoes are lightly browned on top.

9. Let the shepherd's pie cool for 5 minutes before serving.

That's it! Just 5 simple ingredients • ground beef, onion, peas and carrots, mashed potatoes, and seasoning • for a classic and comforting shepherd's pie. You can adjust the amounts of each ingredient to your personal preference.

47. Stuffed Shells: Jumbo pasta shells, ricotta cheese, spinach, marinara sauce, mozzarella.

Ingredient:

- 12 jumbo pasta shells
- 1 cup ricotta cheese
- 2 cups fresh spinach, chopped
- 1 jar (24 oz) marinara sauce
- 1 cup shredded mozzarella cheese

Instructions:

1. Preheat your oven to 375°F.

2. Cook the jumbo pasta shells according to package instructions until al dente. Drain and set aside.

3. In a medium bowl, mix together the ricotta cheese and chopped spinach until well combined.

4. Spread 1/2 cup of the marinara sauce in the bottom of a 9x13 inch baking dish.

5. Stuff each cooked pasta shell with a spoonful of the ricotta•spinach mixture.

6. Arrange the stuffed shells in the baking dish in a single layer.

7. Pour the remaining marinara sauce over the top of the stuffed shells.

8. Sprinkle the shredded mozzarella cheese evenly over the top.

9. Bake for 20•25 minutes, or until the cheese is melted and bubbly.

10. Let the stuffed shells cool for 5 minutes before serving.

That's it! Just 5 simple ingredients • jumbo pasta shells, ricotta cheese, spinach, marinara sauce, and mozzarella • for a delicious and easy stuffed shells dish. You can adjust the amounts of each ingredient to your personal preference.

48. Beef Stroganoff:
Ground beef, egg noodles, sour cream, mushrooms, onion.

Ingredient:

- 1 lb ground beef
- 8 oz egg noodles
- 1 cup sour cream
- 8 oz sliced mushrooms
- 1 onion, diced

Instructions:

1. In a large skillet, cook the ground beef over medium•high heat until browned and crumbled, about 5•7 minutes. Drain any excess fat.

2. Add the diced onion to the skillet and cook for 2•3 minutes, until the onion is translucent.

3. Stir in the sliced mushrooms and cook for an additional 3•4 minutes, until the mushrooms are tender.

4. Meanwhile, cook the egg noodles according to package instructions. Drain and set aside.

5. Reduce the heat to low and stir the sour cream into the beef and vegetable mixture until well combined.

6. Add the cooked egg noodles to the skillet and toss everything together until the noodles are evenly coated.

7. Serve the beef stroganoff immediately, garnished with additional sour cream or chopped parsley if desired.

That's it! Just 5 simple ingredients • ground beef, egg noodles, sour cream, mushrooms, and onion • for a classic and comforting beef stroganoff. You can adjust the amounts of each ingredient to your personal preference.

49. Pulled Pork Sandwich:
Pork shoulder, BBQ sauce, buns, coleslaw mix, pickles.

Ingredient:

- 3 lb pork shoulder (or pork butt)
- 1 cup BBQ sauce
- 8•10 hamburger buns
- 2 cups coleslaw mix
- Dill pickle slices

Instructions:

1. Place the pork shoulder in a slow cooker and cook on low for 8•10 hours, or until the pork is very tender and easily shreds with a fork.

2. Remove the pork from the slow cooker and shred it using two forks. Discard any excess fat.

3. Return the shredded pork to the slow cooker and stir in the BBQ sauce until the pork is evenly coated.

4. To assemble the sandwiches, place a generous portion of the BBQ pulled pork on the bottom half of each hamburger bun.

5. Top the pork with a spoonful of coleslaw mix and a few dill pickle slices.

6. Close the sandwiches with the top buns and serve immediately.

That's it! Just 5 simple ingredients • pork shoulder, BBQ sauce, buns, coleslaw mix, and pickles • for delicious and easy pulled pork sandwiches. You can adjust the amounts of each ingredient to your personal preference.

50. Mushroom Risotto: Arborio rice, mushrooms, chicken broth, Parmesan cheese, onion.

Ingredient:

- 1 cup arborio rice
- 8 oz sliced mushrooms
- 4 cups warm chicken broth
- 1/2 cup grated Parmesan cheese
- 1 onion, diced

Instructions:

1. In a large saucepan, sauté the diced onion in a bit of olive oil over medium heat until translucent, about 3•4 minutes.

2. Add the arborio rice to the pan and stir to coat the grains with the oil. Cook for 2•3 minutes.

3. Ladle in 1 cup of the warm chicken broth and stir constantly until the liquid is absorbed. Repeat this process, adding 1 cup of broth at a time, until the rice is tender and creamy, about 18•22 minutes total.

4. Stir in the sliced mushrooms during the last 5 minutes of cooking to allow them to heat through.

5. Remove the risotto from heat and stir in the grated Parmesan cheese until melted and well combined.

6. Serve the mushroom risotto immediately, garnished with additional Parmesan if desired.

That's it! Just 5 simple ingredients • arborio rice, mushrooms, chicken broth, Parmesan cheese, and onion • for a creamy and flavorful mushroom risotto. You can adjust the amounts of each ingredient to your personal preference.

51. Shrimp Scampi:
Shrimp, garlic, butter, lemon, spaghetti.

Ingredient:

- 1 lb shrimp, peeled and deveined
- 4 cloves garlic, minced
- 4 tbsp unsalted butter
- 1 lemon, juiced
- 8 oz spaghetti

Instructions:

1. Bring a large pot of salted water to a boil. Cook the spaghetti according to package instructions until al dente. Drain and set aside.

2. In a large skillet, melt the butter over medium heat. Add the minced garlic and cook for 1•2 minutes, until fragrant.

3. Add the shrimp to the skillet and cook for 2•3 minutes per side, until the shrimp are pink and opaque.

4. Remove the skillet from heat and stir in the lemon juice.

5. Add the cooked spaghetti to the skillet and toss everything together until the pasta is evenly coated in the garlic•butter sauce.

6. Serve the shrimp scampi immediately, garnished with additional lemon wedges if desired.

That's it! Just 5 simple ingredients • shrimp, garlic, butter, lemon, and spaghetti • for a delicious and easy shrimp scampi dish. You can adjust the amounts of each ingredient to your personal preference.

52. Chicken Marsala:
Chicken breast, Marsala wine, mushrooms, garlic, butter.

Ingredient:

• 4 boneless, skinless chicken breasts
• 1/2 cup Marsala wine
• 8 oz sliced mushrooms
• 3 cloves garlic, minced
• 2 tbsp unsalted butter

Instructions:

1. In a large skillet, melt the butter over medium•high heat.

2. Add the chicken breasts and cook for 4•5 minutes per side, until golden brown. Transfer the chicken to a plate and set aside.

3. Add the sliced mushrooms to the skillet and cook for 3•4 minutes, until they start to soften.

4. Stir in the minced garlic and cook for 1 minute, until fragrant.

5. Pour in the Marsala wine and use a wooden spoon to scrape up any browned bits from the bottom of the pan.

6. Return the chicken breasts to the skillet and simmer for 10•12 minutes, turning the chicken occasionally, until the chicken is cooked through and the sauce has thickened slightly.

7. Serve the Chicken Marsala immediately, spooning the mushroom•wine sauce over the top of the chicken.

That's it! Just 5 simple ingredients • chicken, Marsala wine, mushrooms, garlic, and butter • for a delicious and classic Chicken Marsala dish. You can adjust the amounts of each ingredient to your personal preference.

53. Lentil Soup:
Lentils, carrots, celery, onion, garlic.

Ingredient:

- 1 cup dried lentils, rinsed
- 3 carrots, peeled and diced
- 2 stalks celery, diced
- 1 onion, diced
- 3 cloves garlic, minced

Instructions:

1. In a large pot, combine the rinsed lentils, diced carrots, diced celery, diced onion, and minced garlic.

2. Add 4 cups of water or low•sodium vegetable broth to the pot.

3. Bring the soup to a boil over high heat, then reduce the heat to medium•low and let it simmer for 20•25 minutes, or until the lentils are tender.

4. Season the soup with salt and pepper to taste.

5. Serve the lentil soup hot, garnished with chopped parsley or a drizzle of olive oil if desired.

That's it! Just 5 simple ingredients • lentils, carrots, celery, onion, and garlic • for a nourishing and flavorful lentil soup. You can adjust the amounts of each ingredient to your personal preference.

Some variations could include:
- Adding diced tomatoes
- Using a different type of broth (chicken or beef)
- Stirring in a splash of lemon juice or red wine vinegar at the end
- Topping with crumbled feta or shredded cheese

54. Beef Tacos:
Ground beef, taco seasoning, tortillas, lettuce, cheese.

Ingredient:

- 1 lb ground beef
- 2 tbsp taco seasoning
- 8•10 small tortillas (corn or flour)
- 1 cup shredded lettuce
- 1 cup shredded cheese (cheddar or Mexican blend)

Instructions:

1. In a large skillet, cook the ground beef over medium•high heat until browned and crumbled, about 5•7 minutes. Drain any excess fat.

2. Sprinkle the taco seasoning over the cooked ground beef and stir to coat the meat evenly.

3. Warm the tortillas according to package instructions, either in a dry skillet or wrapped in a damp paper towel and microwaved for 30 seconds.

4. To assemble the tacos, place a spoonful of the seasoned ground beef in the center of each tortilla.

5. Top the beef with shredded lettuce and shredded cheese.

6. Serve the beef tacos immediately, with any additional toppings or condiments on the side.

That's it! Just 5 simple ingredients • ground beef, taco seasoning, tortillas, lettuce, and cheese • for delicious and customizable beef tacos. You can adjust the amounts of each ingredient to your personal preference.

55. Chicken Parmesan: Chicken breast, marinara sauce, mozzarella, Parmesan, breadcrumbs.

Ingredient:

- 4 boneless, skinless chicken breasts
- 1 cup marinara sauce
- 1 cup shredded mozzarella cheese
- 1/2 cup grated Parmesan cheese
- 1 cup breadcrumbs

Instructions:

1. Preheat your oven to 400°F.

2. Pound the chicken breasts lightly to an even thickness, about 1/2 inch thick.

3. In a shallow dish, combine the breadcrumbs and grated Parmesan cheese.

4. Dredge the chicken breasts in the breadcrumb mixture, coating both sides.

5. Place the breaded chicken in a baking dish.

6. Top each chicken breast with a few tablespoons of marinara sauce, followed by the shredded mozzarella cheese.

7. Bake for 20•25 minutes, until the chicken is cooked through and the cheese is melted and bubbly.

8. Serve the Chicken Parmesan immediately, with extra marinara sauce on the side if desired.

That's it! Just 5 simple ingredients • chicken, marinara sauce, mozzarella, Parmesan, and breadcrumbs • for a classic and delicious Chicken Parmesan dish. You can adjust the amounts of each ingredient to your personal preference.

56. Fish Tacos:
White fish, tortillas, cabbage, lime, salsa.

Ingredient:

• 1 lb white fish fillets (such as tilapia, cod, or halibut), cut into 1•inch pieces
• 8•10 small corn or flour tortillas
• 2 cups shredded cabbage
• 1 lime, cut into wedges
• 1 cup salsa

Instructions:

1. In a large skillet, cook the fish pieces over medium•high heat for 3•4 minutes per side, until the fish is opaque and flakes easily with a fork.

2. Warm the tortillas according to package instructions, either in a dry skillet or wrapped in a damp paper towel and microwaved for 30 seconds.

3. To assemble the tacos, place a few pieces of the cooked fish in the center of each warm tortilla.

4. Top the fish with a generous amount of shredded cabbage.

5. Serve the fish tacos immediately, with the lime wedges and salsa on the side for guests to add as desired.

That's it! Just 5 simple ingredients • white fish, tortillas, cabbage, lime, and salsa • for delicious and easy fish tacos. You can adjust the amounts of each ingredient to your personal preference.

57. Cabbage Rolls:
Cabbage, ground beef, rice, tomato sauce, onion.

Ingredient:

- 1 head of green cabbage
- 1 lb ground beef
- 1 cup cooked rice
- 1 (15 oz) can tomato sauce
- 1 onion, diced

Instructions:

1. Bring a large pot of water to a boil. Carefully add the whole head of cabbage and cook for 5•7 minutes, until the outer leaves are softened. Remove the cabbage from the water and let it cool slightly.

2. In a bowl, mix together the ground beef, cooked rice, and diced onion until well combined.

3. Carefully peel the softened cabbage leaves off the head, keeping them intact. Place a spoonful of the beef and rice mixture onto the center of each leaf.

4. Fold the sides of the leaf over the filling, then roll up the leaf tightly to enclose the filling.

5. Arrange the stuffed cabbage rolls seam•side down in a baking dish. Pour the tomato sauce over the top.

6. Bake the cabbage rolls at 375°F for 45•60 minutes, until the cabbage is tender and the filling is cooked through.

That's it! Just 5 simple ingredients • cabbage, ground beef, rice, tomato sauce, and onion • for delicious and comforting cabbage rolls. You can adjust the amounts of each ingredient to your personal preference.

Let me know if you need any clarification on the recipe!

58. Vegetable Curry:
Potatoes, carrots, peas, coconut milk, curry powder.

Ingredient:
- 2 medium potatoes, peeled and cubed
- 2 carrots, peeled and sliced
- 1 cup frozen peas
- 1 (13.5 oz) can coconut milk
- 2 tbsp curry powder

Instructions:

1. In a large saucepan or Dutch oven, combine the cubed potatoes, sliced carrots, and frozen peas.

2. Pour in the can of coconut milk and sprinkle the curry powder over the top.

3. Stir everything together until the curry powder is well distributed.

4. Bring the mixture to a boil over high heat, then reduce the heat to medium•low and let it simmer for 15•20 minutes, or until the potatoes and carrots are tender.

5. Taste and adjust the seasoning as needed, adding more curry powder for a stronger flavor.

6. Serve the vegetable curry hot, over rice if desired.

That's it! Just 5 simple ingredients • potatoes, carrots, peas, coconut milk, and curry powder • for a flavorful and easy vegetable curry. You can adjust the amounts of each ingredient to your personal preference.

Some variations could include:
- Adding diced onion or garlic
- Using a different type of vegetable (such as cauliflower or spinach)
- Substituting the coconut milk with vegetable or chicken broth

59. Burrito Bowl:
Rice, black beans, chicken, salsa, cheese.

Ingredient:

- 1 cup cooked rice
- 1 (15 oz) can black beans, drained and rinsed
- 1 lb cooked chicken, shredded or diced
- 1 cup salsa
- 1 cup shredded cheese (cheddar or Mexican blend)

Instructions:

1. In a large bowl, layer the cooked rice on the bottom.

2. Top the rice with the drained and rinsed black beans.

3. Add the cooked and shredded or diced chicken on top of the beans.

4. Spoon the salsa over the chicken.

5. Sprinkle the shredded cheese evenly over the top.

6. Serve the burrito bowl immediately, or refrigerate until ready to serve.

You can customize the burrito bowl by adding other toppings like diced avocado, sour cream, chopped cilantro, or diced onion.

That's it! Just 5 simple ingredients • rice, black beans, chicken, salsa, and cheese • for a delicious and easy burrito bowl. You can adjust the amounts of each ingredient to your personal preference.

60. Pork Chops:
Pork chops, apples, cinnamon, brown sugar, butter.

Ingredient:

- 4 pork chops
- 2 apples, peeled, cored and sliced
- 2 tbsp brown sugar
- 1 tsp ground cinnamon
- 2 tbsp butter

Instructions:

1. Season the pork chops with salt and pepper.

2. In a large skillet over medium•high heat, melt the butter. Add the pork chops and cook for 3•4 minutes per side until browned.

3. Add the apple slices, brown sugar, and cinnamon to the skillet. Stir to coat the apples.

4. Reduce heat to medium•low, cover and cook for 10•15 minutes, turning the pork chops occasionally, until the pork is cooked through and the apples are tender.

5. Serve the pork chops topped with the cinnamon•sugar apples.

Enjoy your simple 5•ingredient pork chop dinner!

61. Fruit Salad:
Strawberries, blueberries, kiwi, pineapple, mint.

Ingredient:

- 1 lb fresh strawberries, hulled and halved
- 1 cup fresh blueberries
- 2 kiwi fruits, peeled and sliced
- 1 cup diced fresh pineapple
- 1/4 cup fresh mint leaves, chopped

Instructions:

1. In a large bowl, gently combine the strawberries, blueberries, kiwi, and pineapple.

2. Sprinkle the chopped mint over the top.

3. Toss the fruit salad gently to mix everything together.

4. Serve immediately or refrigerate until ready to serve. The fruit salad is best enjoyed within 1•2 days.

The combination of sweet berries, tart kiwi, and refreshing pineapple and mint makes this a delightful and healthy fruit salad. Adjust the amounts of each fruit to your taste preferences. Enjoy!

62. Guacamole:
Avocado, lime, red onion, tomato, cilantro.

Ingredient:

• 3 ripe avocados, pitted and diced
• 2 tablespoons freshly squeezed lime juice
• 1/4 cup finely diced red onion
• 1 Roma tomato, diced
• 2 tablespoons chopped fresh cilantro
• 1/2 teaspoon salt
• 1/4 teaspoon ground black pepper

Instructions:

1. In a medium bowl, gently mash the avocado chunks with a fork, leaving some small chunks.

2. Stir in the lime juice, red onion, tomato, cilantro, salt, and pepper. Mix well to combine.

3. Taste and adjust seasoning as needed, adding more lime juice for acidity, salt for flavor, or cilantro for freshness.

4. Serve immediately with tortilla chips, or cover surface with plastic wrap to prevent browning and refrigerate until ready to serve.

The key to great guacamole is using ripe, creamy avocados and balancing the flavors of the lime, onion, tomato, and cilantro. Adjust the amounts of each ingredient to suit your personal taste preferences. Enjoy this classic guacamole dip!

63. Veggie Sticks with Hummus:
Carrots, celery, bell peppers, cucumbers, hummus.

Ingredient:
- 1 cup baby carrots
- 1 cup celery sticks
- 1 cup bell pepper strips (any color)
- 1 cup cucumber slices
- 1 cup prepared hummus

Instructions:

1. Wash and prepare the vegetables:
- Peel and cut the carrots into sticks
- Slice the celery into sticks
- Slice the bell peppers into strips
- Slice the cucumber into rounds or sticks

2. Arrange the vegetable sticks on a platter or in individual serving dishes.

3. Place the hummus in a small bowl in the center of the platter.

4. Serve the veggie sticks alongside the hummus for dipping.

That's it! This simple 5•ingredient snack or appetizer provides a nutritious and flavorful combination of fresh vegetables and creamy hummus. The variety of crunchy veggies pairs perfectly with the smooth, savory hummus. Adjust the amounts of each vegetable to your taste preferences.

Enjoy this easy, healthy, and delicious veggie and hummus platter!

64. Yogurt and Honey:
Greek yogurt, honey, walnuts, cinnamon, bananas.

Ingredient:

- 2 cups plain Greek yogurt
- 2 tbsp honey
- 1/4 cup chopped walnuts
- 1 tsp ground cinnamon
- 1 banana, sliced

Instructions:

1. In a bowl, combine the Greek yogurt and honey. Stir until the honey is fully incorporated.

2. Top the yogurt mixture with the chopped walnuts and ground cinnamon.

3. Arrange the sliced banana on top of the yogurt.

4. Serve immediately or refrigerate until ready to serve.

That's it! Just 5 simple ingredients • Greek yogurt, honey, walnuts, cinnamon, and banana • for a delicious and healthy yogurt parfait.

You can adjust the amounts of each ingredient to your personal preference. Some variations could include:

- Using different types of nuts (such as almonds or pecans)
- Adding a drizzle of maple syrup or honey on top
- Sprinkling granola or crushed graham crackers over the top
- Substituting the banana with other fresh fruit (berries, mango, etc.)

65. Popcorn:
Popcorn kernels, butter, salt, Parmesan cheese, garlic powder.

Ingredient:

- 1/2 cup popcorn kernels
- 2 tablespoons butter, melted
- 1/2 teaspoon salt
- 1/4 cup grated Parmesan cheese
- 1/2 teaspoon garlic powder

Instructions:

1. Pop the popcorn kernels according to package instructions, either on the stovetop or in the microwave.

2. In a large bowl, drizzle the melted butter over the freshly popped popcorn and toss to coat.

3. Sprinkle the salt, Parmesan cheese, and garlic powder over the buttered popcorn. Toss again to evenly distribute the seasonings.

4. Serve the Parmesan garlic popcorn warm and enjoy!

That's it • just 5 simple ingredients to make this flavorful and satisfying popcorn snack. The combination of savory Parmesan, garlic, and butter complements the popcorn perfectly.

You can adjust the amounts of each seasoning to suit your taste preferences. For example, add more or less salt, Parmesan, or garlic powder depending on your personal flavor preferences.

This Parmesan garlic popcorn makes a great movie night snack or party appetizer. Enjoy!

66. Cheese and Crackers:
Cheese, crackers, grapes, almonds, fig jam.

Ingredient:

• Assorted cheese (such as cheddar, brie, gouda)
• Assorted crackers
• Grapes
• Almonds
• Fig jam

Instructions:

1. Arrange the cheese, crackers, grapes, and almonds on a serving platter or board.

2. Place small spoonfuls of the fig jam around the platter.

That's it! This 5•ingredient cheese and crackers snack is easy to put together and makes a great appetizer or light meal.

The key is to choose a variety of cheese flavors and textures, such as a firm cheddar, a soft brie, and a semi•hard gouda. Pair them with different types of crackers, from crisp water crackers to hearty whole grain crackers.

The grapes and almonds add freshness and crunch, while the fig jam provides a sweet and tangy complement to the cheese.

Feel free to adjust the amounts of each ingredient to suit your tastes and the number of people you're serving. This is a very flexible and customizable snack platter. Enjoy!

67. Ants on a Log:
Celery, peanut butter, raisins, sunflower seeds, honey.

Ingredient:

- Celery stalks, cut into 3•4 inch pieces
- Peanut butter
- Raisins
- Sunflower seeds
- Honey (optional)

Instructions:

1. Wash and cut the celery stalks into 3•4 inch pieces.

2. Spread peanut butter into the "trough" of the celery pieces.

3. Top the peanut butter with raisins, to resemble "ants" on the "log" (celery).

4. Sprinkle sunflower seeds over the top.

5. Drizzle a small amount of honey over the top, if desired.

That's it! This simple, 5•ingredient snack is a classic kids' treat. The combination of crunchy celery, creamy peanut butter, sweet raisins, and crunchy sunflower seeds makes for a tasty and nutritious snack. Enjoy!

68. Fruit and Nut Mix: Almonds, cashews, raisins, dried cranberries, dark chocolate chips.

Ingredient:

- 1 cup raw almonds
- 1 cup raw cashews
- 1 cup raisins
- 1 cup dried cranberries
- 1/2 cup dark chocolate chips

Instructions:

1. In a large bowl, combine the almonds, cashews, raisins, dried cranberries, and dark chocolate chips.

2. Stir the ingredients together until well mixed.

3. Transfer the fruit and nut mix to an airtight container or resealable bag.

That's it! This 5•ingredient mix makes a great healthy snack or trail mix. The combination of nuts, dried fruit, and dark chocolate provides a balance of protein, healthy fats, fiber, and antioxidants. Feel free to adjust the ratios of each ingredient to your taste preferences.

Store the fruit and nut mix in an airtight container at room temperature for up to 2 weeks. Enjoy as a quick snack or sprinkle over yogurt, oatmeal, or salads.

69. Avocado and Tomato Salad:
Avocado, cherry tomatoes, lime juice, red onion, cilantro.

Ingredient:

• 2 avocados, diced
• 1 pint cherry tomatoes, halved
• 1/4 cup diced red onion
• 2 tbsp fresh lime juice
• 2 tbsp chopped fresh cilantro

Instructions:

1. In a large bowl, gently combine the diced avocado and halved cherry tomatoes.

2. Add the diced red onion, fresh lime juice, and chopped cilantro.

3. Toss the salad ingredients together until everything is evenly coated.

4. Season with salt and pepper to taste.

5. Serve the avocado and tomato salad immediately, or refrigerate until ready to serve.

That's it! Just 5 simple ingredients • avocado, cherry tomatoes, red onion, lime juice, and cilantro • for a fresh and flavorful salad.

You can adjust the amounts of each ingredient to your personal preference. Some variations could include:

• Adding a drizzle of olive oil
• Substituting the lime juice with balsamic vinegar
• Sprinkling crumbled feta or queso fresco on top
• Serving the salad on a bed of mixed greens

70. Apple Slices with Peanut Butter:
Apple, peanut butter, honey, cinnamon, granola.

Ingredient:

- 2 apples, cored and sliced
- 1/2 cup creamy peanut butter
- 2 tablespoons honey
- 1/2 teaspoon ground cinnamon
- 1/4 cup granola

Instructions:

1. Wash and core the apples, then slice them into wedges or rounds.

2. In a small bowl, mix together the peanut butter and honey until well combined.

3. Arrange the apple slices on a serving plate or platter.

4. Drizzle the peanut butter•honey mixture over the apple slices, using a spoon to spread it evenly.

5. Sprinkle the ground cinnamon and granola over the top of the peanut butter•coated apples.

That's it! This simple 5•ingredient snack or dessert is a delicious and nutritious way to enjoy apples.

The creamy peanut butter and sweet honey complement the crisp apples, while the cinnamon and crunchy granola add warmth and texture.

You can adjust the amounts of each ingredient to your taste preferences. For example, use more or less peanut butter, honey, cinnamon, or granola.

This apple and peanut butter snack is perfect for a healthy treat, after•school snack, or light dessert. Enjoy!

71. Cucumber Bites:
Cucumber, cream cheese, smoked salmon, dill, lemon zest.

Ingredient:

• 1 English cucumber, sliced into 1/2•inch thick rounds
• 4 oz cream cheese, softened
• 4 oz smoked salmon, thinly sliced
• 2 tablespoons chopped fresh dill
• 1 teaspoon lemon zest

Instructions:

1. Slice the cucumber into 1/2•inch thick rounds and arrange them on a serving platter.

2. In a small bowl, mix together the softened cream cheese, chopped dill, and lemon zest until well combined.

3. Top each cucumber round with a small dollop of the cream cheese mixture.

4. Tear or cut the smoked salmon into small pieces and place a piece on top of the cream cheese on each cucumber bite.

5. Garnish with an extra sprig of fresh dill, if desired.

That's it! These 5•ingredient cucumber bites make a refreshing and elegant appetizer or snack. The cool, crisp cucumber pairs perfectly with the creamy cheese, salty smoked salmon, and bright flavors of dill and lemon.

You can adjust the amounts of each ingredient to your taste preferences. For example, use more or less cream cheese, salmon, dill, or lemon zest depending on your personal flavor profile.

These cucumber bites are easy to assemble and make a beautiful presentation. Enjoy this simple yet delicious recipe!

72. Deviled Eggs:
Eggs, mayonnaise, mustard, paprika, pickles.

Ingredient:

• 6 hard•boiled eggs, peeled
• 2 tablespoons mayonnaise
• 1 teaspoon Dijon mustard
• 1/4 teaspoon paprika, plus more for garnish
• 1 tablespoon finely chopped dill pickles

Instructions:

1. Slice the hard•boiled eggs in half lengthwise and carefully remove the yolks, placing them in a small bowl.

2. In the bowl with the yolks, mash them with a fork. Add the mayonnaise, Dijon mustard, and paprika. Mix until well combined and creamy.

3. Spoon or pipe the yolk mixture back into the egg white halves.

4. Sprinkle the tops of the deviled eggs with a light dusting of additional paprika.

5. Top each deviled egg with a small piece of chopped dill pickle.

That's it! These classic 5•ingredient deviled eggs are a simple yet delicious appetizer or snack.

The creamy yolk mixture gets its flavor from the mayonnaise, mustard, and paprika. The dill pickle adds a nice tangy crunch on top.

You can customize the deviled eggs by adjusting the amounts of mayonnaise, mustard, or paprika to your taste preferences. You can also try adding other seasonings like garlic powder, chives, or a dash of hot sauce.

Serve these deviled eggs chilled or at room temperature. Enjoy this easy and crowd•pleasing appetizer!

73. Rice Cakes with Toppings: Rice cakes, avocado, cherry tomatoes, smoked salmon, arugula.

Ingredient:

• 4 whole grain rice cakes
• 1 ripe avocado, mashed
• 1 cup cherry tomatoes, halved
• 4 oz smoked salmon, flaked
• 1 cup baby arugula leaves

Instructions:

1. Spread the mashed avocado evenly over the surface of the rice cakes.

2. Top each rice cake with a portion of the cherry tomato halves.

3. Sprinkle the flaked smoked salmon over the tomatoes.

4. Finish by arranging a small handful of baby arugula leaves on top of each rice cake.

That's it! This simple 5•ingredient rice cake creation makes for a nutritious and flavorful snack or light meal.

The creamy avocado, juicy tomatoes, savory smoked salmon, and peppery arugula all come together beautifully on the crisp rice cake base.

You can adjust the amounts of each topping to your personal taste preferences. For example, use more or less avocado, salmon, tomatoes, or arugula.

These rice cake bites are easy to assemble and make a great healthy option for a quick breakfast, lunch, or snack. Enjoy!

74. Mini Quesadillas:
Tortillas, cheese, black beans, salsa, avocado.

Ingredient:

• 8 small flour tortillas (4•5 inches in diameter)
• 1 cup shredded cheese (cheddar, Monterey Jack, or Mexican blend)
• 1 (15 oz) can black beans, drained and rinsed
• 1 cup salsa
• 1 avocado, diced

Instructions:

1. Preheat a skillet or griddle over medium heat.

2. Place one tortilla in the skillet. Sprinkle 2•3 tablespoons of shredded cheese over half of the tortilla.

3. Top the cheese with 2•3 tablespoons of black beans, a spoonful of salsa, and a few pieces of diced avocado.

4. Fold the tortilla in half to create a half•moon shape. Cook for 2•3 minutes per side, until the cheese is melted and the tortilla is lightly browned.

5. Repeat with the remaining tortillas and fillings to make 8 mini quesadillas.

6. Serve the mini quesadillas warm, with extra salsa and avocado on the side for dipping.

That's it! These 5•ingredient mini quesadillas are a quick and easy appetizer or snack. The combination of melty cheese, black beans, salsa, and avocado is so flavorful.

You can customize the fillings to your liking, using different types of cheese, beans, or toppings. Enjoy these tasty mini quesadillas!

75. Chocolate•Dipped Strawberries:
Strawberries, dark chocolate, coconut oil, sea salt, pistachios.

Ingredient:

- 12 fresh strawberries, washed and patted dry
- 4 oz dark chocolate, chopped
- 1 tablespoon coconut oil
- 1/4 teaspoon sea salt
- 2 tablespoons chopped pistachios

Instructions:

1. Line a baking sheet with parchment paper.

2. In a double boiler or microwave, melt the chopped dark chocolate and coconut oil together, stirring frequently until smooth.

3. One at a time, dip the strawberries into the melted chocolate mixture, coating them about 3/4 of the way up.

4. Gently tap off any excess chocolate and place the dipped strawberries on the prepared baking sheet.

5. Sprinkle a small pinch of sea salt over each chocolate•dipped strawberry.

6. Lastly, sprinkle the chopped pistachios over the top of the strawberries.

7. Refrigerate the chocolate•dipped strawberries for at least 30 minutes to allow the chocolate to set.

That's it! These 5•ingredient chocolate•dipped strawberries are a decadent and elegant treat.

The dark chocolate and coconut oil create a smooth, shiny coating, while the sea salt and chopped pistachios add a delightful crunch and salty•sweet contrast.

You can customize this recipe by using different types of chocolate, nuts, or even drizzling the set strawberries with additional melted chocolate.

Enjoy these chocolate•dipped strawberries as a dessert, snack, or even an edible gift. They're sure to impress!

76. Chocolate Chip Cookies:
Flour, butter, sugar, eggs, chocolate chips.

Ingredient:

- 2 cups all•purpose flour
- 1 cup unsalted butter, softened
- 1 cup granulated sugar
- 2 large eggs
- 1 cup semi•sweet chocolate chips

Instructions:

1. Preheat your oven to 375°F. Line a baking sheet with parchment paper.

2. In a medium bowl, whisk together the flour. Set aside.

3. In a large bowl, beat the softened butter and sugar together until light and fluffy, about 2•3 minutes. Beat in the eggs one at a time until fully incorporated.

4. Gradually mix the dry flour mixture into the wet ingredients until just combined. Fold in the chocolate chips.

5. Scoop rounded tablespoons of dough onto the prepared baking sheet, spacing them about 2 inches apart.

6. Bake for 10•12 minutes, until the edges are lightly golden brown.

7. Allow the cookies to cool on the baking sheet for 5 minutes before transferring to a wire rack to cool completely.

That's it! These simple 5•ingredient chocolate chip cookies are a classic treat. The combination of butter, sugar, eggs, flour, and chocolate chips creates a deliciously soft and chewy cookie.

You can customize the cookies by using different types of chocolate chips, adding nuts, or even rolling the dough in cinnamon•sugar before baking. Adjust the baking time as needed to achieve your desired cookie texture.

Enjoy these homemade chocolate chip cookies warm or at room temperature. They make a great snack or dessert!

77. Brownies:
Cocoa powder, flour, butter, sugar, eggs.

Ingredient:

- 1/2 cup (1 stick) unsalted butter, melted
- 1 cup granulated sugar
- 2 large eggs
- 1/2 cup all•purpose flour
- 1/3 cup unsweetened cocoa powder

Instructions:

1. Preheat your oven to 350°F. Grease an 8x8 inch baking pan.

2. In a medium bowl, whisk together the melted butter and sugar until combined.

3. Beat in the eggs one at a time, mixing well after each addition.

4. Sift in the flour and cocoa powder, then use a rubber spatula to gently fold the dry ingredients into the wet ingredients until just combined (do not overmix).

5. Spread the brownie batter evenly into the prepared baking pan.

6. Bake for 20•25 minutes, until a toothpick inserted in the center comes out with just a few moist crumbs attached.

7. Allow the brownies to cool completely in the pan before cutting into squares.

That's it! These rich, fudgy 5•ingredient brownies are a classic and easy•to•make dessert.

The combination of melted butter, sugar, eggs, flour, and cocoa powder creates a dense, chocolatey brownie with a crackly top.

You can customize the brownies by adding chopped nuts, chocolate chips, or a sprinkle of sea salt on top. Adjust the baking time as needed to achieve your desired level of fudginess.

Enjoy these homemade brownies on their own or with a scoop of vanilla ice cream. They're sure to satisfy any chocolate craving!

78. Banana Bread:
Bananas, flour, sugar, eggs, baking soda.

Ingredient:

• 3 ripe bananas, mashed (about 1 cup)
• 1 1/2 cups all•purpose flour
• 3/4 cup granulated sugar
• 2 large eggs
• 1 teaspoon baking soda

Instructions:

1. Preheat your oven to 350°F. Grease a 9x5 inch loaf pan.

2. In a medium bowl, mash the ripe bananas until smooth.

3. In a separate bowl, whisk together the flour, sugar, and baking soda.

4. Add the eggs to the mashed bananas and mix until well combined.

5. Pour the banana mixture into the dry ingredients and stir just until no dry pockets remain (do not overmix).

6. Scrape the batter into the prepared loaf pan and smooth the top.

7. Bake for 55•65 minutes, until a toothpick inserted in the center comes out clean.

8. Allow the banana bread to cool in the pan for 10 minutes, then transfer to a wire rack to cool completely before slicing.

That's it! This 5•ingredient banana bread is moist, flavorful, and so easy to make.

The ripe bananas provide natural sweetness, while the flour, sugar, eggs, and baking soda create the perfect quick bread texture.

You can customize the banana bread by adding chopped nuts, chocolate chips, or a streusel topping. Adjust the baking time as needed based on your oven.

Enjoy this classic homemade banana bread for breakfast, snack, or dessert. It's sure to become a family favorite!

79. Pancake Muffins:
Pancake mix, milk, eggs, blueberries, maple syrup.

Ingredient:

- 1 cup pancake mix
- 3/4 cup milk
- 2 eggs
- 1 cup fresh or frozen blueberries
- 2 tablespoons maple syrup

Instructions:

1. Preheat your oven to 350°F. Grease a 12•cup muffin tin.

2. In a medium bowl, whisk together the pancake mix, milk, and eggs until just combined (do not overmix).

3. Gently fold the blueberries into the pancake batter.

4. Spoon the batter evenly into the prepared muffin cups, filling them about 3/4 full.

5. Bake for 15•18 minutes, until the muffins are golden brown and a toothpick inserted in the center comes out clean.

6. Drizzle the warm pancake muffins with maple syrup before serving.

That's it! These 5•ingredient pancake muffins are a fun and easy breakfast or brunch option. The blueberries add pops of juicy sweetness throughout the fluffy pancake batter.

You can customize the muffins by using different types of berries, chocolate chips, or nuts. Adjust the amount of maple syrup to your taste preference as well.

Serve these pancake muffins warm, with extra maple syrup on the side for drizzling. Enjoy this simple yet delicious breakfast treat!

80. Apple Crisp:
Apples, oats, butter, cinnamon, brown sugar.

Ingredient:

• 6 cups peeled, cored, and sliced apples (about 6•8 medium apples)
• 1 cup old•fashioned rolled oats
• 1/2 cup unsalted butter, cubed
• 1/2 cup packed brown sugar
• 1 teaspoon ground cinnamon

Instructions:

1. Preheat your oven to 350°F. Grease an 8x8 inch baking dish.

2. Arrange the sliced apples in an even layer in the prepared baking dish.

3. In a medium bowl, combine the rolled oats, cubed butter, brown sugar, and cinnamon. Use your fingers to mix and crumble the mixture until it resembles coarse crumbs.

4. Sprinkle the oat topping evenly over the apples.

5. Bake for 30•35 minutes, until the apples are tender and the topping is golden brown.

6. Allow the apple crisp to cool for 10•15 minutes before serving.

That's it! This 5•ingredient apple crisp is a classic and comforting dessert.

The tender, cinnamon•spiced apples are topped with a buttery, crumbly oat topping that gets perfectly crisp in the oven.

You can customize the apple crisp by using different types of apples, adding nuts or raisins to the topping, or serving it with a scoop of vanilla ice cream.

Enjoy this easy and delicious apple crisp warm, at room temperature, or chilled. It's the perfect fall or winter treat!

81. Rice Pudding:
Rice, milk, sugar, vanilla extract, cinnamon.

Ingredient:

• 1 cup uncooked short•grain white rice
• 4 cups whole milk
• 1/2 cup granulated sugar
• 1 teaspoon vanilla extract
• 1/2 teaspoon ground cinnamon

Instructions:

1. In a medium saucepan, combine the uncooked rice and milk. Bring to a gentle simmer over medium heat, stirring occasionally.

2. Once simmering, reduce the heat to low and continue cooking, stirring frequently, for 30•40 minutes, until the rice is very soft and the mixture has thickened to a creamy, pudding•like consistency.

3. Remove the pan from the heat and stir in the sugar and vanilla extract until fully incorporated.

4. Transfer the rice pudding to a serving bowl or individual ramekins. Sprinkle the top with the ground cinnamon.

5. Serve the rice pudding warm, at room temperature, or chilled, depending on your preference.

That's it! This 5•ingredient rice pudding is a classic, comforting dessert.

The combination of plump, creamy rice, rich milk, sweet sugar, and aromatic vanilla and cinnamon creates a delightfully smooth and satisfying pudding.

You can customize the rice pudding by using different types of milk (such as almond or coconut milk), adding dried fruit, or topping it with toasted nuts or a drizzle of honey.

Enjoy this simple, homemade rice pudding as a cozy, old•fashioned treat. It's perfect for breakfast, dessert, or anytime you need a comforting sweet indulgence.

82. Peanut Butter Cookies:
Peanut butter, sugar, egg, vanilla extract, baking soda.

Ingredient:

• 1 cup creamy peanut butter
• 1 cup granulated sugar
• 1 large egg
• 1 teaspoon vanilla extract
• 1/2 teaspoon baking soda

Instructions:

1. Preheat your oven to 350°F. Line a baking sheet with parchment paper.

2. In a medium bowl, stir together the peanut butter, sugar, egg, vanilla, and baking soda until well combined. The dough will be thick.

3. Scoop rounded tablespoons of dough and place them about 2 inches apart on the prepared baking sheet.

4. Use a fork to gently press a criss•cross pattern into the top of each cookie dough ball, flattening them slightly.

5. Bake for 8•10 minutes, until the cookies are lightly golden around the edges.

6. Allow the cookies to cool on the baking sheet for 5 minutes before transferring them to a wire rack to cool completely.

That's it! These 5•ingredient peanut butter cookies are a classic and easy•to•make treat.

The combination of peanut butter, sugar, egg, vanilla, and baking soda creates a soft, chewy, and peanut•y cookie. The fork marks on top give them a classic look.

You can customize the cookies by using crunchy peanut butter, adding chocolate chips, or rolling the dough in sugar before baking. Adjust the baking time as needed to achieve your desired texture.

Enjoy these homemade peanut butter cookies as a snack, dessert, or even for gift•giving. They're sure to satisfy any peanut butter craving!

83. Chocolate Mousse:
Chocolate, eggs, sugar, heavy cream, vanilla extract.

Ingredient:

- 6 oz dark chocolate, chopped
- 3 large eggs, separated
- 1/4 cup granulated sugar
- 1 cup heavy whipping cream
- 1 teaspoon vanilla extract

Instructions:

1. In a medium heatproof bowl, melt the chopped chocolate either over a double boiler or in the microwave, stirring frequently until smooth. Allow to cool slightly.

2. In a large bowl, beat the egg yolks and 2 tablespoons of the sugar until light and fluffy.

3. In a separate bowl, beat the egg whites with the remaining 2 tablespoons of sugar until stiff peaks form.

4. In another bowl, whip the heavy cream with the vanilla extract until soft peaks form.

5. Gently fold the whipped cream into the melted chocolate until combined.

6. Fold in the beaten egg yolks, then gently fold in the whipped egg whites.

7. Spoon or pipe the chocolate mousse into individual serving dishes. Refrigerate for at least 2 hours before serving.

That's it! This 5•ingredient chocolate mousse is rich, airy, and decadent.

The combination of melted chocolate, egg yolks, whipped cream, and whipped egg whites creates a luxuriously smooth and creamy texture. The vanilla adds a lovely flavor.

You can customize the mousse by using different types of chocolate or adding a splash of liqueur. Garnish with shaved chocolate, cocoa powder, or fresh berries before serving.

Enjoy this easy and impressive homemade chocolate mousse as a special dessert. It's sure to impress!

84. Fruit Tart:
Pie crust, pastry cream, strawberries, kiwi, blueberries.

Ingredient:

- 1 pre•made pie crust
- 1 cup prepared pastry cream
- 1 cup sliced strawberries
- 1 kiwi, peeled and sliced
- 1 cup fresh blueberries

Instructions:

1. Preheat your oven to 375°F. Press the pie crust into a 9•inch tart pan with a removable bottom. Prick the bottom with a fork.

2. Bake the pie crust for 12•15 minutes, until lightly golden. Allow it to cool completely.

3. Spread the prepared pastry cream evenly over the cooled tart crust.

4. Arrange the sliced strawberries, kiwi, and blueberries in a decorative pattern over the top of the pastry cream.

5. Refrigerate the fruit tart for at least 2 hours before serving to allow the filling to set.

That's it! This 5•ingredient fruit tart is a simple yet elegant dessert.

The buttery pie crust provides a sturdy base for the creamy pastry cream and fresh, colorful fruit topping. You can use any combination of seasonal berries and stone fruits that you prefer.

For best results, use a pre•made pie crust to save time. The pastry cream can also be made in advance.

Serve this chilled fruit tart as a light and refreshing dessert. Enjoy!

85. Cheesecake Bites:
Cream cheese, sugar, eggs, vanilla extract, graham cracker crust.

Ingredient:

- 16 oz cream cheese, softened
- 1/2 cup granulated sugar
- 2 large eggs
- 1 teaspoon vanilla extract
- 1 cup graham cracker crumbs

Instructions:

1. Preheat your oven to 325°F. Grease a 24•cup mini muffin tin.

2. In a large bowl, beat the softened cream cheese with an electric mixer until smooth and creamy.

3. Add the sugar, eggs, and vanilla extract. Beat until well combined and the mixture is light and fluffy.

4. Sprinkle 1•2 tablespoons of graham cracker crumbs into the bottom of each muffin cup.

5. Spoon or pipe the cheesecake batter evenly into the muffin cups, filling them about 3/4 full.

6. Bake for 18•20 minutes, until the centers are just set.

7. Allow the cheesecake bites to cool completely in the muffin tin before removing them.

8. Once cooled, gently remove the cheesecake bites from the tin and serve.

That's it! These 5•ingredient cheesecake bites are a simple and delicious no•bake dessert.

The creamy cheesecake filling paired with the crunchy graham cracker crust makes for a perfect bite•sized treat. You can top the bites with fresh fruit, caramel, or chocolate if desired.

Store any leftover cheesecake bites in the refrigerator for up to 5 days. Enjoy this easy and crowd•pleasing dessert!

86. Lemon Bars:
Lemon juice, sugar, flour, butter, eggs.

Ingredient:

• 1/2 cup (1 stick) unsalted butter, melted
• 1 cup all•purpose flour
• 1 cup granulated sugar
• 3 large eggs
• 1/2 cup freshly squeezed lemon juice (about 2•3 lemons)

Instructions:

For the Crust:
1. Preheat the oven to 350°F. Grease an 8x8 inch baking pan.
2. In a medium bowl, stir together the melted butter and flour until a dough forms.
3. Press the dough evenly into the bottom of the prepared baking pan.
4. Bake for 15 minutes.

For the Lemon Filling:
1. In a medium bowl, whisk together the sugar, eggs, and lemon juice until well combined.
2. Pour the lemon filling over the hot crust.
3. Bake for an additional 20•25 minutes, until the filling is set.
4. Allow the lemon bars to cool completely in the pan before cutting into squares.

That's it! These 5•ingredient lemon bars have a buttery shortbread crust and a tangy, creamy lemon filling.

The combination of fresh lemon juice, sugar, eggs, and a touch of flour creates the perfect balance of sweet and tart.

You can dust the cooled lemon bars with powdered sugar before serving, if desired. Adjust the amount of lemon juice to your personal taste preference.

These easy lemon bars are a refreshing and crowd•pleasing dessert. Enjoy!

87. Pumpkin Pie:
Pumpkin puree, sugar, eggs, condensed milk, pie crust.

Ingredient:

- 1 (15 oz) can pumpkin puree
- 1 cup granulated sugar
- 2 large eggs
- 1 (12 oz) can evaporated milk
- 1 pre•made 9•inch pie crust

Instructions:

1. Preheat your oven to 425°F.

2. In a large bowl, whisk together the pumpkin puree, sugar, eggs, and evaporated milk until well combined.

3. Pour the pumpkin pie filling into the pre•made pie crust.

4. Bake for 15 minutes at 425°F, then reduce the oven temperature to 350°F and continue baking for 40•50 minutes, until the center is almost set.

5. Allow the pumpkin pie to cool completely, at least 2•3 hours, before slicing and serving.

6. Optionally, you can serve the pumpkin pie chilled or at room temperature, with whipped cream or vanilla ice cream.

That's it! This 5•ingredient pumpkin pie is a classic and easy•to•make dessert.

The combination of pumpkin puree, sugar, eggs, and evaporated milk creates a rich, creamy, and perfectly spiced filling. The pre•made pie crust makes this recipe super simple.

You can customize the pumpkin pie by adding a sprinkle of cinnamon, nutmeg, or ginger to the filling. You can also make your own homemade pie crust if desired.

Enjoy this classic pumpkin pie as a delicious Thanksgiving or holiday dessert. It's sure to be a crowd•pleaser!

88. Pineapple Upside•Down Cake:
Pineapple, cake mix, brown sugar, butter, cherries.

Ingredient:

• 1 (20 oz) can pineapple slices, drained (reserve 2 tablespoons of the pineapple juice)
• 1 (15.25 oz) box yellow cake mix
• 1/2 cup packed brown sugar
• 1/4 cup unsalted butter, melted
• 10•12 maraschino cherries, halved

Instructions:

1. Preheat your oven to 350°F. Grease a 9•inch round baking pan.

2. Arrange the pineapple slices in a single layer in the bottom of the prepared pan. Place a maraschino cherry half in the center of each pineapple slice.

3. In a medium bowl, combine the yellow cake mix, 2 tablespoons of the reserved pineapple juice, and the melted butter. Stir until just combined (do not overmix).

4. Sprinkle the brown sugar evenly over the pineapple slices.

5. Carefully pour the cake batter over the brown sugar and pineapple.

6. Bake for 40•45 minutes, until a toothpick inserted in the center comes out clean.

7. Allow the cake to cool in the pan for 10 minutes, then invert it onto a serving plate.

Serve the pineapple upside•down cake warm or at room temperature. Enjoy!

This 5•ingredient cake is a classic and easy•to•make dessert. The caramelized brown sugar and pineapple create a delicious topping, while the moist yellow cake base completes the dish.

You can customize the cake by using different types of fruit, adding nuts, or even drizzling it with a glaze. Adjust the baking time as needed for your oven.

This pineapple upside•down cake is sure to be a hit at any gathering. Enjoy this retro and delicious dessert!

89. Chocolate Fondue:
Chocolate, heavy cream, strawberries, marshmallows, bananas.

Ingredient:

- 12 oz semisweet chocolate, chopped
- 1 cup heavy cream
- 1 cup fresh strawberries, halved
- 1 cup mini marshmallows
- 1 banana, sliced

Instructions:

1. In a medium saucepan, heat the heavy cream over medium heat, stirring occasionally, until it just begins to simmer.

2. Remove the pan from the heat and add the chopped chocolate. Let it sit for 2•3 minutes to allow the chocolate to melt.

3. Whisk the chocolate and cream together until smooth and fully combined, creating a rich, creamy fondue.

4. Transfer the chocolate fondue to a fondue pot or small slow cooker set to the warm setting to keep it melted and smooth.

5. Arrange the strawberries, marshmallows, and banana slices around the fondue pot for dipping.

6. Serve the chocolate fondue warm, with skewers or fondue forks for dipping the fruit and marshmallows.

That's it! This 5•ingredient chocolate fondue is a classic and indulgent dessert.

The combination of melted semisweet chocolate and heavy cream creates a luxuriously smooth and rich fondue. The fresh fruit and marshmallows provide the perfect dippers.

You can customize the fondue by using different types of chocolate, adding a splash of liqueur, or including other dipping items like pound cake, pretzels, or graham crackers.

Enjoy this easy and impressive chocolate fondue as a fun, interactive dessert for parties or special occasions. It's sure to be a crowd•pleaser!

90. Caramel Apples:
Apples, caramel, nuts, chocolate, sprinkles.

Ingredient:
• 6 medium•sized apples, washed and dried
• 1 cup prepared caramel sauce
• 1/2 cup chopped nuts (such as peanuts, pecans, or almonds)
• 1/2 cup melted chocolate (milk, dark, or white)
• Sprinkles or crushed cookies (optional)

Instructions:
1. Insert a popsicle stick or wooden skewer into the stem end of each apple.

2. In a shallow bowl or plate, pour the prepared caramel sauce.

3. One at a time, dip each apple into the caramel sauce, turning to coat the entire surface. Allow any excess caramel to drip off.

4. Place the caramel•coated apples on a parchment•lined baking sheet or plate.

5. Sprinkle the chopped nuts over the caramel•coated apples, pressing them gently to adhere.

6. Drizzle the melted chocolate over the top of the caramel apples.

7. If desired, sprinkle the apples with additional toppings like sprinkles or crushed cookies.

8. Refrigerate the caramel apples for at least 30 minutes to allow the caramel and chocolate to set.

That's it! These 5•ingredient caramel apples are a classic and delicious fall treat.

The combination of crisp apples, gooey caramel, crunchy nuts, and rich chocolate makes for an irresistible dessert or snack. You can customize the toppings to your liking.

Be sure to use a high•quality caramel sauce for best results. You can also make your own homemade caramel if desired.

Enjoy these decadent caramel apples as a fun and festive dessert or gift. They're sure to impress!

91. Peach Cobbler:
Peaches, sugar, flour, butter, cinnamon.

Ingredient:

• 4 cups sliced fresh or canned peaches
• 1 cup granulated sugar
• 1 cup all•purpose flour
• 1/2 cup unsalted butter, melted
• 1 teaspoon ground cinnamon

Instructions:

1. Preheat your oven to 375°F. Grease a 9x13 inch baking dish.

2. Arrange the sliced peaches in an even layer in the prepared baking dish.

3. In a medium bowl, whisk together the sugar, flour, and cinnamon.

4. Drizzle the melted butter over the peaches, then sprinkle the flour•sugar mixture evenly over the top.

5. Bake for 30•35 minutes, until the topping is golden brown and the peaches are bubbly.

6. Allow the peach cobbler to cool for 10•15 minutes before serving.

7. Serve warm, optionally with a scoop of vanilla ice cream or whipped cream.

That's it! This 5•ingredient peach cobbler is a classic and comforting dessert.

The sweet, juicy peaches are topped with a simple flour•sugar•cinnamon topping that bakes up into a delicious, golden crust. The melted butter helps create a nice crisp texture.

You can use fresh, canned, or frozen peaches for this recipe. Adjust the amount of sugar based on the sweetness of your peaches.

Enjoy this easy and delicious peach cobbler as a perfect summer or fall dessert. It's sure to be a crowd•pleaser!

92. Ice Cream Sandwiches:
Cookies, ice cream, chocolate chips, sprinkles, whipped cream.

Ingredient:
- 12 chocolate chip cookies (or your favorite cookie)
- 1 pint of your favorite ice cream, softened
- 1/2 cup mini chocolate chips
- 1/4 cup rainbow sprinkles
- 1 cup whipped cream (optional)

Instructions:

1. Line a baking sheet with parchment paper.

2. Place 6 of the cookies face•down on the prepared baking sheet. Scoop about 1/4 cup of the softened ice cream onto each cookie and spread it out evenly.

3. Top each ice cream•topped cookie with another cookie, pressing down gently to adhere.

4. Sprinkle the mini chocolate chips and rainbow sprinkles over the top of the ice cream sandwiches.

5. Freeze the ice cream sandwiches for at least 2 hours, until firm.

6. If desired, top the frozen ice cream sandwiches with a dollop of whipped cream just before serving.

That's it! These 5•ingredient homemade ice cream sandwiches are a fun and delicious treat.

The combination of chewy cookies, creamy ice cream, and crunchy toppings makes for a perfect summertime dessert. You can use any flavor of ice cream and cookies that you prefer.

For best results, work quickly when assembling the sandwiches to prevent the ice cream from melting. Store any leftover ice cream sandwiches in the freezer.

Enjoy these easy and customizable homemade ice cream sandwiches as a refreshing and indulgent dessert!

93. Tiramisu:
Ladyfingers, coffee, mascarpone, cocoa powder, sugar.

Ingredient:

- 1 package (about 24) ladyfinger cookies
- 1 cup strong brewed coffee, cooled
- 1 lb mascarpone cheese
- 1/2 cup granulated sugar
- 2 tablespoons unsweetened cocoa powder

Instructions:

1. In a shallow bowl, pour the cooled coffee. Quickly dip half of the ladyfingers into the coffee, coating both sides. Arrange the soaked ladyfingers in a single layer in an 8x8 inch baking dish.

2. In a medium bowl, beat the mascarpone and sugar together until smooth and creamy.

3. Spread half of the mascarpone mixture evenly over the ladyfingers in the baking dish.

4. Repeat the layers, dipping and arranging the remaining ladyfingers, then topping with the remaining mascarpone mixture.

5. Dust the top of the tiramisu evenly with the cocoa powder.

6. Cover and refrigerate the tiramisu for at least 6 hours, or up to 24 hours, before serving.

That's it! This 5•ingredient tiramisu is a classic Italian dessert with layers of coffee•soaked ladyfingers and creamy mascarpone.

The combination of the rich mascarpone, strong coffee, and bitter cocoa powder creates a wonderfully balanced and indulgent treat.

You can customize the tiramisu by using different types of liqueurs or extracts in the coffee, or by adding a layer of chocolate shavings or chopped nuts.

Chill the tiramisu thoroughly before serving for the best texture and flavor. Enjoy this easy and impressive no•bake dessert!

94. Panna Cotta: Heavy cream, sugar, vanilla extract, gelatin, berries.

Ingredient:

• 2 cups heavy cream
• 1/4 cup granulated sugar
• 1 teaspoon vanilla extract
• 1 packet (about 1 tablespoon) unflavored gelatin powder
• 1 cup mixed fresh berries (such as raspberries, blackberries, and blueberries)

Instructions:

1. In a medium saucepan, combine the heavy cream and sugar. Heat over medium, stirring occasionally, until the sugar has dissolved and the mixture is hot but not boiling.

2. Remove the cream mixture from the heat and stir in the vanilla extract.

3. In a small bowl, sprinkle the gelatin powder over 2 tablespoons of cold water. Let it sit for 5 minutes to bloom.

4. Whisk the bloomed gelatin into the hot cream mixture until fully dissolved.

5. Divide the panna cotta mixture evenly between 4•6 ramekins or small bowls. Refrigerate for at least 4 hours, or until set.

6. When ready to serve, run a knife around the edge of each panna cotta and invert onto a plate. Top with the fresh mixed berries.

That's it! This 5•ingredient panna cotta is a light, creamy, and elegant Italian dessert.

The combination of rich heavy cream, sweet sugar, and floral vanilla is set with just a touch of gelatin for a silky smooth texture. The fresh berries provide a bright, refreshing contrast.

You can customize the panna cotta by using different types of cream, adding citrus zest or liqueur, or topping it with other seasonal fruits.

Enjoy this easy and impressive no•bake dessert chilled, as a light and sophisticated end to any meal.

95. Berry Parfait:
Berries, Greek yogurt, honey, granola, mint.

Ingredient:

• 1 cup mixed berries (such as strawberries, blueberries, raspberries)
• 1 cup plain Greek yogurt
• 2 tablespoons honey
• 1/2 cup granola
• Fresh mint leaves for garnish

Instructions:

1. In a parfait glass or small bowl, layer the ingredients in the following order:
   • 1/4 cup berries
   • 1/4 cup Greek yogurt
   • 1 teaspoon honey
   • 2 tablespoons granola
   • Repeat the layers until you reach the top of the glass.

2. Top with a sprig of fresh mint.

3. Serve chilled.

The combination of sweet berries, tangy Greek yogurt, crunchy granola, and fresh mint creates a delightful and healthy parfait. Adjust the amounts of each ingredient to your taste preferences. Enjoy!

96. Mango Sorbet: Mango, sugar, lime juice, water, mint.

Ingredient:

- 2 cups chopped ripe mango (about 2•3 mangoes)
- 1/2 cup granulated sugar
- 2 tablespoons fresh lime juice
- 1/4 cup water
- Fresh mint leaves for garnish

Instructions:

1. In a blender or food processor, puree the chopped mango until smooth.

2. In a small saucepan, combine the sugar and water. Heat over medium, stirring occasionally, until the sugar has fully dissolved. Allow the simple syrup to cool completely.

3. In a medium bowl, stir together the mango puree, lime juice, and the cooled simple syrup until well combined.

4. Pour the mango mixture into an ice cream maker and churn according to the manufacturer's instructions, usually 20•30 minutes, until thickened and frozen.

5. Transfer the mango sorbet to an airtight container and freeze for at least 2 hours before serving.

6. Scoop the sorbet into serving dishes and garnish with fresh mint leaves.

The bright, sweet•tart flavor of the mango sorbet is perfectly complemented by the fresh lime juice and cooling mint. Enjoy this refreshing and flavorful frozen treat!

97. Fudgesicles:
Cocoa powder, milk, sugar, cornstarch, vanilla extract.

Ingredient:

- 1/4 cup unsweetened cocoa powder
- 1/4 cup granulated sugar
- 2 tablespoons cornstarch
- 1/8 teaspoon salt
- 2 cups milk (any type)
- 1 teaspoon vanilla extract

Instructions:

1. In a medium saucepan, whisk together the cocoa powder, sugar, cornstarch, and salt until well combined.

2. Gradually whisk in the milk, making sure there are no lumps.

3. Place the saucepan over medium heat and cook, stirring constantly, until the mixture thickens and comes to a gentle boil, about 5•7 minutes.

4. Remove from heat and stir in the vanilla extract.

5. Carefully pour the hot chocolate mixture into popsicle molds or small paper cups. Insert popsicle sticks.

6. Freeze for at least 4 hours, or until completely set.

7. To remove the fudgesicles, run the molds under warm water for 30 seconds to 1 minute, then gently pull the popsicles out.

The cornstarch helps create a rich, creamy fudge•like texture, while the cocoa powder and vanilla provide the classic fudgesicle flavor. Enjoy these homemade frozen treats!

98. Banana Ice Cream:
Frozen bananas, peanut butter, cocoa powder, milk, vanilla extract.

Ingredient:

• 3•4 ripe bananas, peeled and frozen
• 2 tbsp peanut butter
• 2 tbsp cocoa powder
• 1/4 cup milk (dairy, almond, or oat milk)
• 1 tsp vanilla extract

Instructions:

1. Add the frozen banana chunks, peanut butter, cocoa powder, milk, and vanilla extract to a high•powered blender or food processor.

2. Blend or process the ingredients until smooth and creamy, scraping down the sides as needed. The mixture should have an ice cream•like texture.

3. Serve immediately for a soft serve consistency, or transfer to an airtight container and freeze for 2•3 hours for a firmer ice cream texture.

4. Scoop and enjoy your homemade Banana Ice Cream! Top with extra peanut butter, chocolate chips, nuts, or your favorite toppings.

The frozen bananas provide the base, while the peanut butter, cocoa powder, milk, and vanilla create a rich, creamy, and chocolatey flavor. This is a simple, healthy, and delicious frozen treat.

99. Raspberry Cheesecake:
Cream cheese, sugar, eggs, raspberries, graham cracker crust.

Ingredient:

Crust:
• 1 1/2 cups graham cracker crumbs
• 5 tbsp unsalted butter, melted

Filling:
• 24 oz (3 packages) cream cheese, softened
• 1 cup granulated sugar
• 3 large eggs
• 1 tsp vanilla extract
• 1 cup fresh or frozen raspberries

Instructions:

Crust:
1. Preheat oven to 325°F. Grease a 9•inch springform pan.
2. In a medium bowl, mix together the graham cracker crumbs and melted butter until well combined.
3. Press the mixture firmly into the bottom and slightly up the sides of the prepared springform pan.
4. Bake for 8 minutes, then let cool completely.

Filling:
1. In a large bowl, beat the cream cheese with an electric mixer until light and fluffy, about 2•3 minutes.
2. Gradually add in the sugar and beat until smooth, scraping down the sides as needed.
3. Add the eggs one at a time, beating well after each addition. Mix in the vanilla.
4. Gently fold in the raspberries, being careful not to overmix.
5. Pour the cheesecake batter into the prepared crust.
6. Bake for 55•65 minutes, until the center is almost set.
7. Turn off the oven and let the cheesecake remain in the oven for 1 hour.
8. Remove from oven and let cool completely on a wire rack, then refrigerate for at least 4 hours or overnight before serving.

Enjoy this creamy, tangy raspberry cheesecake with the sweet graham cracker crust!

100. Chocolate Truffles: Chocolate, heavy cream, cocoa powder, vanilla extract, sea salt.

Ingredient:

• 8 oz high•quality dark chocolate, chopped
• 1/2 cup heavy cream
• 1 tsp vanilla extract
• 1/4 tsp sea salt
• Cocoa powder, for coating

Instructions:

1. Place the chopped chocolate in a medium heatproof bowl.

2. In a small saucepan, heat the heavy cream over medium heat until it just begins to simmer. Remove from heat and pour the hot cream over the chocolate. Let sit for 2•3 minutes to allow the chocolate to melt.

3. Whisk the chocolate and cream together until smooth and fully combined. Stir in the vanilla extract and sea salt.

4. Cover the bowl and refrigerate the chocolate mixture for 1•2 hours, until firm enough to scoop.

5. Using a small cookie scoop or spoon, scoop out tablespoon•sized portions of the chocolate mixture and roll them into smooth balls between your palms.

6. Roll the truffles in cocoa powder to coat completely.

7. Store the truffles in an airtight container in the refrigerator for up to 1 week. Enjoy chilled.

The rich dark chocolate, creamy ganache, and touch of salt make these homemade truffles absolutely decadent. They make a wonderful homemade gift or treat.

101. Strawberry Shortcake:
Biscuits, strawberries, sugar, whipped cream, vanilla extract.

Ingredient:

For the Biscuits:
• 2 cups all•purpose flour
• 2 teaspoons baking powder
• 1/2 teaspoon salt
• 5 tablespoons unsalted butter, chilled and cubed
• 3/4 cup cold milk

For the Strawberries:
• 1 lb fresh strawberries, hulled and sliced
• 2•3 tablespoons granulated sugar

For the Whipped Cream:
• 1 cup heavy whipping cream
• 2 tablespoons powdered sugar
• 1 teaspoon vanilla extract

Instructions:

1. Make the Biscuits:
   • Preheat oven to 450°F. Line a baking sheet with parchment paper.
   • In a large bowl, whisk together the flour, baking powder, and salt. Cut in the chilled butter using a pastry cutter or two forks until mixture resembles coarse crumbs.
   • Slowly pour in the cold milk and stir just until a shaggy dough forms. Do not overmix.
   • Turn dough onto a lightly floured surface and gently knead 2•3 times. Pat into a 3/4•inch thick round.
   • Use a 2•inch biscuit cutter to cut out biscuits, pressing straight down without twisting. Place on the prepared baking sheet.
   • Bake for 12•15 minutes, until golden brown on top.

2. Make the Strawberries:
   • In a medium bowl, gently toss the sliced strawberries with 2•3 tablespoons of sugar. Let sit for 15 minutes to macerate.

3. Make the Whipped Cream:
   • In a large bowl, beat the heavy cream with a hand mixer until soft peaks form. Add the powdered sugar and vanilla and continue beating until stiff peaks form.

4. Assemble the Shortcake:
   • Split the warm biscuits in half horizontally. Top the bottom halves with the macerated strawberries and their juices.
   • Dollop the whipped cream over the strawberries.
   • Place the top biscuit halves over the whipped cream.
   • Serve immediately.

Enjoy this classic summertime dessert with the sweet, juicy strawberries, fluffy biscuits, and fresh whipped cream!

102. Nutella Crepes:
Crepes, Nutella, bananas, powdered sugar, strawberries.

Ingredient:

For the Crepes:
• 1 cup all•purpose flour
• 2 eggs
• 1 cup milk
• 2 tablespoons unsalted butter, melted, plus more for cooking
• 1/4 teaspoon salt

For the Filling:
• 1/2 cup Nutella (or other chocolate•hazelnut spread)
• 1 banana, sliced
• Powdered sugar, for dusting
• Fresh strawberries, sliced (optional)

Instructions:

1. Make the Crepe Batter:
   • In a medium bowl, whisk together the flour, eggs, milk, 2 tablespoons melted butter, and salt until smooth. Let the batter rest for 30 minutes.

2. Cook the Crepes:
   • Heat a 8•inch non•stick skillet or crepe pan over medium heat. Lightly grease the pan with butter.
   • Pour about 1/4 cup of the batter into the pan, tilting and swirling to evenly coat the bottom.
   • Cook for 1•2 minutes, until the edges start to lift and the center is set. Flip and cook for another 30 seconds to 1 minute.
   • Transfer the crepe to a plate and cover to keep warm. Repeat with the remaining batter, greasing the pan as needed.

3. Assemble the Crepes:
   • Spread about 2 tablespoons of Nutella down the center of each crepe.
   • Top with sliced banana.
   • Fold the crepe in half, then in half again to form a triangle.

4. Serve:
   • Arrange the filled crepes on a serving plate.
   • Dust with powdered sugar and top with sliced strawberries, if desired.
   • Serve immediately while warm.

103. Cinnamon Rolls:
Dough, cinnamon, sugar, butter, cream cheese frosting.

Ingredient:

- 3/4 cup warm milk
- 2 1/4 teaspoons active dry yeast (1 standard packet)
- 1/4 cup granulated sugar
- 1/4 cup unsalted butter, melted
- 1 large egg
- 1/2 teaspoon salt
- 4 cups all•purpose flour, plus more for dusting

Filling Ingredients:
- 1/2 cup unsalted butter, softened
- 1 cup brown sugar
- 2 tablespoons ground cinnamon

Cream Cheese Frosting Ingredients:
- 4 ounces cream cheese, softened
- 1/4 cup unsalted butter, softened
- 1 1/2 cups powdered sugar
- 1/2 teaspoon vanilla extract
- 1/8 teaspoon salt

Instructions:

1. Make the Dough:
   • In a medium bowl, combine the warm milk, yeast, and 1 tablespoon of the sugar. Let sit for 5•10 minutes until foamy.
   • In a large bowl, whisk together the remaining sugar, melted butter, egg, and salt.
   • Add the yeast mixture and 3 cups of the flour. Mix until a shaggy dough forms.
   • Turn the dough out onto a lightly floured surface and knead for 5•7 minutes, adding more flour as needed, until the dough is smooth and elastic.
   • Place the dough in a lightly greased bowl, cover, and let rise for 1 hour or until doubled in size.

2. Make the Filling:
   • In a small bowl, mix together the softened butter, brown sugar, and cinnamon until well combined.

3. Assemble the Cinnamon Rolls:
   • Punch down the risen dough to release air bubbles. Roll out on a lightly floured surface into a 12x18•inch rectangle.
   • Spread the cinnamon•sugar filling evenly over the dough, leaving a 1/2•inch border.
   • Tightly roll up the dough from the long side to form a log. Slice into 12 equal pieces.
   • Place the rolls in a greased 9x13•inch baking dish. Cover and let rise for 30 minutes.

4. Bake the Cinnamon Rolls:
   • Preheat oven to 350°F.
   • Bake the rolls for 20•25 minutes, until golden brown.

104. Peach Galette:
Pie crust, peaches, sugar, flour, butter.

Ingredient:

For the Crust:
• 1 1/4 cups all•purpose flour
• 1 tablespoon granulated sugar
• 1/4 teaspoon salt
• 8 tablespoons (1 stick) unsalted butter, chilled and cubed
• 3•5 tablespoons ice water

For the Filling:
• 4•5 ripe peaches, pitted and sliced 1/4•inch thick
• 1/4 cup granulated sugar
• 2 tablespoons all•purpose flour
• 1 tablespoon unsalted butter, cubed

For Finishing:
• 1 egg, beaten with 1 tablespoon water (for egg wash)
• 1 tablespoon coarse sugar (optional)

Instructions:

1. Make the Crust:
   • In a food processor, pulse the flour, sugar, and salt to combine. Add the chilled butter cubes and pulse until the mixture resembles coarse crumbs with some pea•sized pieces of butter remaining.
   • Add the ice water 1 tablespoon at a time, pulsing just until the dough begins to hold together. Do not overmix.
   • Turn the dough out onto a lightly floured surface and gather into a disk. Wrap in plastic wrap and refrigerate for at least 1 hour.

2. Make the Filling:
   • In a medium bowl, gently toss the sliced peaches with the sugar and flour until evenly coated.

3. Assemble the Galette:
   • Preheat oven to 400°F. Line a baking sheet with parchment paper.
   • On a lightly floured surface, roll the chilled dough into a 12•inch circle, about 1/8•inch thick. Transfer to the prepared baking sheet.
   • Arrange the peach slices in the center of the dough, leaving a 2•inch border. Fold the dough over the peaches, pleating it as you go.
   • Dot the peaches with the cubed butter.

4. Bake the Galette:
   • Brush the dough with the egg wash and sprinkle with coarse sugar, if desired.
   • Bake for 35•40 minutes, until the crust is golden brown and the peaches are tender.
   • Allow to cool for 10 minutes before slicing and serving.

105. Cherry Clafoutis:
Cherries, eggs, milk, sugar, flour.

Ingredient:

• 1 lb fresh cherries, pitted
• 3 large eggs
• 1 cup whole milk
• 1/2 cup granulated sugar
• 1/3 cup all•purpose flour
• 1/4 teaspoon salt
• Powdered sugar for dusting

Instructions:

1. Preheat the oven to 350°F. Grease a 9•inch pie dish or baking dish.

2. Arrange the pitted cherries in an even layer in the prepared baking dish.

3. In a medium bowl, whisk together the eggs, milk, granulated sugar, flour, and salt until smooth and well combined.

4. Pour the egg mixture over the cherries, making sure they are evenly coated.

5. Bake for 35•40 minutes, until the center is set and the top is lightly golden brown.

6. Allow the clafoutis to cool for at least 15 minutes before serving.

7. Dust the top generously with powdered sugar just before serving.

Tips:
• You can use other types of fruit, such as plums, apples, or berries, in place of the cherries.
• For a richer texture, use half•and•half or heavy cream instead of milk.
• Add a teaspoon of vanilla extract or almond extract to the batter.
• Serve the clafoutis warm or at room temperature.

The classic French dessert, clafoutis, features a soft, custard•like batter surrounding sweet, juicy cherries. It's simple to make but impressive to serve. Enjoy this delightful cherry•studded treat!

106. Lemonade:
Lemons, water, sugar, mint, ice.

Ingredient:

• 6 lemons, juiced (about 1 cup fresh lemon juice)
• 1 cup granulated sugar
• 4 cups cold water
• Fresh mint leaves for garnish
• Ice cubes

Instructions:

1. Make the Lemon Simple Syrup:
   • In a small saucepan, combine the sugar and 1 cup of water. Bring to a simmer over medium heat, stirring occasionally, until the sugar has fully dissolved. Remove from heat and let cool completely.

2. Prepare the Lemonade:
   • In a large pitcher, stir together the lemon juice, the cooled simple syrup, and the remaining 3 cups of cold water until well combined.

3. Serve the Lemonade:
   • Fill glasses with ice cubes.
   • Pour the lemonade over the ice.
   • Garnish each glass with a fresh mint sprig.

Variations:
• For a sweeter lemonade, add more simple syrup to taste.
• For a less sweet lemonade, use less simple syrup or add more lemon juice.
• Try adding sliced lemons, limes, or strawberries to the pitcher for extra flavor and color.
• Spike it with vodka or gin for an adult version.

This homemade lemonade is refreshing, tangy, and perfectly sweetened. The simple syrup helps the sugar fully dissolve for a smooth, balanced flavor. Enjoy this classic summertime drink!

107. Iced Coffee:
Coffee, milk, sugar, ice, vanilla extract.

Ingredient:

- 1 cup freshly brewed strong coffee, cooled
- 1 cup cold milk (dairy, almond, oat, etc.)
- 2•3 tablespoons granulated sugar (or to taste)
- 1/2 teaspoon vanilla extract
- Ice cubes

Instructions:

1. In a pitcher or large glass, stir together the cooled coffee, milk, sugar, and vanilla extract until the sugar has dissolved.

2. Fill a glass with ice cubes.

3. Pour the iced coffee over the ice.

4. Stir gently and serve immediately.

Variations:
- Use sweetened condensed milk instead of regular milk for a creamier, richer iced coffee.
- Add a splash of chocolate syrup or caramel sauce for a mocha or caramel iced coffee.
- Blend the iced coffee with ice for a frappuccino•style drink.
- Top with whipped cream, chocolate shavings, or a sprinkle of cinnamon.
- Make it an iced coffee cocktail by adding a shot of liquor like rum, Kahlua, or Irish cream.

The key to great iced coffee is starting with a strong, freshly brewed coffee. Adjust the sugar and milk to your personal taste preferences. This easy homemade version is perfect for hot summer days or anytime you need a refreshing caffeine boost.

108. Smoothie:
Banana, spinach, almond milk, peanut butter, honey.

Ingredient:

- 1 ripe banana, frozen
- 1 cup fresh spinach leaves
- 1 cup unsweetened almond milk
- 2 tablespoons creamy peanut butter
- 1 tablespoon honey

Instructions:

1. Add the frozen banana, spinach, almond milk, peanut butter, and honey to a high•powered blender.

2. Blend on high speed until the mixture is smooth and creamy, about 1•2 minutes.

3. Scrape down the sides of the blender as needed to ensure all ingredients are fully incorporated.

4. Pour the smoothie into a glass and enjoy immediately.

Optional Variations:
- Add a scoop of vanilla protein powder for extra protein.
- Use Greek yogurt instead of almond milk for a thicker, creamier texture.
- Swap the peanut butter for almond butter or cashew butter.
- Add a handful of ice cubes for a chilled, frosty smoothie.
- Top with extra banana slices, granola, or a sprinkle of cinnamon.

This nutrient•dense smoothie is a great way to start the day or enjoy as a healthy snack. The banana and peanut butter provide natural sweetness, while the spinach adds a boost of vitamins and minerals. Adjust the ingredient amounts to suit your taste preferences.

109. Hot Chocolate:
Cocoa powder, milk, sugar, vanilla extract, marshmallows.

Ingredient:
- 2 cups milk (dairy, almond, oat, etc.)
- 2 tablespoons unsweetened cocoa powder
- 2 tablespoons granulated sugar
- 1/4 teaspoon vanilla extract
- Pinch of salt
- Marshmallows for topping (optional)

Instructions:

1. In a small saucepan, whisk together the milk, cocoa powder, sugar, vanilla, and salt.

2. Heat the mixture over medium heat, whisking frequently, until it just begins to steam and bubble around the edges. Do not boil.

3. Remove the saucepan from the heat and continue whisking for 1•2 minutes to ensure the cocoa powder and sugar are fully dissolved.

4. Pour the hot chocolate into mugs.

5. Top with marshmallows, if desired.

Variations:
- For a richer hot chocolate, use half•and•half or heavy cream instead of milk.
- Add a pinch of cinnamon, nutmeg, or cayenne pepper for a spiced hot chocolate.
- Stir in a tablespoon of peanut butter or Nutella for a decadent twist.
- Top with whipped cream, chocolate shavings, or a drizzle of caramel sauce.
- Make it an adult beverage by adding a shot of liquor like Kahlua, Bailey's, or peppermint schnapps.

This homemade hot chocolate is creamy, chocolatey, and perfectly sweetened. The vanilla and pinch of salt help to balance the flavors. Enjoy this cozy, comforting drink on a chilly day.

110. Green Tea Lemonade:
Green tea, lemon juice, honey, water, ice.

Ingredient:

• 4 green tea bags
• 4 cups boiling water
• 1/2 cup freshly squeezed lemon juice (about 3•4 lemons)
• 1/4 cup honey, or to taste
• Ice cubes

Instructions:

1. Steep the green tea bags in the boiling water for 3•5 minutes. Remove the tea bags and let the tea cool to room temperature.

2. In a pitcher, stir together the brewed green tea, lemon juice, and honey until the honey is fully dissolved.

3. Taste and adjust sweetness as needed, adding more honey if desired.

4. Fill glasses with ice cubes.

5. Pour the green tea lemonade over the ice.

6. Garnish with lemon slices, if desired.

Variations:
• Use matcha powder instead of green tea bags for a more intense green tea flavor.
• Add a splash of sparkling water or club soda for a fizzy twist.
• Muddle some fresh mint leaves in the bottom of the glasses before pouring in the lemonade.
• Substitute agave nectar or maple syrup for the honey.
• For an adult version, stir in a shot of vodka or gin.

The combination of bright, tangy lemon and the earthy, grassy notes of green tea creates a refreshing and hydrating beverage. Adjust the sweetness to your personal taste. Enjoy this healthy and flavorful iced tea lemonade!

111. Mango Lassi:
Mango, yogurt, sugar, water, cardamom.

Ingredient:

• 2 cups chopped ripe mango (about 2 medium mangoes)
• 1 cup plain yogurt
• 1/4 cup water
• 2•3 tablespoons granulated sugar, to taste
• 1/4 teaspoon ground cardamom
• Ice cubes (optional)

Instructions:

1. In a blender, combine the chopped mango, yogurt, water, sugar, and cardamom. Blend until smooth and creamy.

2. Taste and adjust the sweetness as needed, adding more sugar if desired.

3. If a thinner consistency is preferred, add a bit more water and blend again.

4. Fill glasses with ice cubes (optional).

5. Pour the mango lassi into the glasses.

6. Garnish with a slice of fresh mango or a sprinkle of ground cardamom, if desired.

Variations:
• Use plain Greek yogurt for a thicker, creamier lassi.
• Add a splash of rose water or a pinch of saffron for an aromatic twist.
• Substitute honey or maple syrup for the sugar.
• Blend in a handful of ice cubes for a chilled, frothy lassi.
• Top with toasted coconut flakes or crushed pistachios.

The mango lassi is a refreshing and creamy Indian•inspired drink that combines the sweetness of ripe mangoes with the tanginess of yogurt. Adjust the sugar and cardamom to your taste preferences. Enjoy this delightful summer beverage!

112. Berry Smoothie:
Mixed berries, yogurt, honey, milk, ice.

Ingredient:

• 1 cup mixed berries (such as strawberries, blueberries, raspberries, blackberries)
• 1 cup plain Greek yogurt
• 1/2 cup milk (dairy, almond, oat, etc.)
• 2 tablespoons honey (or to taste)
• 1 cup ice cubes

Instructions:

1. In a blender, combine the mixed berries, Greek yogurt, milk, and honey.

2. Add the ice cubes and blend on high speed until the mixture is smooth and creamy, about 1•2 minutes.

3. Taste and adjust sweetness as needed, adding more honey if desired.

4. Pour the berry smoothie into glasses and serve immediately.

Variations:
• Use frozen berries instead of fresh for a thicker, colder smoothie.
• Add a handful of spinach or kale for extra nutrients.
• Substitute plain yogurt for vanilla or fruit•flavored yogurt.
• Include a scoop of protein powder or nut butter for extra protein.
• Top with fresh berries, granola, or a drizzle of honey.

This berry smoothie is a delicious and nutritious way to start the day or enjoy as a refreshing snack. The combination of sweet berries, tangy yogurt, and creamy milk creates a well•balanced flavor. Adjust the ingredients to your taste preferences.

113. Arnold Palmer:
Iced tea, lemonade, sugar, lemon slices, ice.

Ingredient:

• 1 cup freshly brewed iced tea, chilled
• 1 cup freshly squeezed lemonade, chilled
• 1•2 tablespoons granulated sugar (optional)
• Lemon slices for garnish
• Ice cubes

Instructions:

1. In a pitcher or large glass, combine the chilled iced tea and lemonade.

2. Stir in the sugar, if using, until dissolved.

3. Fill glasses with ice cubes.

4. Pour the Arnold Palmer over the ice.

5. Garnish each glass with a lemon slice.

Variations:
• Use unsweetened iced tea and adjust the sugar to your taste preference.
• Try different types of tea, such as black, green, or herbal.
• Add a splash of club soda or sparkling water for a fizzy twist.
• Muddle some fresh mint leaves in the bottom of the glasses before pouring.
• For an adult version, stir in a shot of vodka or gin.

The Arnold Palmer is a classic refreshing beverage that combines the tartness of lemonade with the subtle bitterness of iced tea. It's the perfect thirst•quenching drink for hot summer days. Adjust the ratio of tea to lemonade to suit your personal taste.

114. Orange Julius:
Orange juice, milk, sugar, vanilla extract, ice.

Ingredient:
• 1 cup fresh orange juice (about 3•4 oranges)
• 1 cup milk (dairy, almond, or oat)
• 2 tablespoons granulated sugar
• 1 teaspoon vanilla extract
• 1 cup ice cubes

Instructions:

1. In a blender, combine the orange juice, milk, sugar, and vanilla extract.

2. Add the ice cubes and blend on high speed until smooth and frothy, about 1•2 minutes.

3. Taste and adjust sweetness as needed, adding more sugar if desired.

4. Pour the Orange Julius into glasses.

Variations:
• Use frozen orange juice concentrate instead of fresh orange juice.
• Substitute half•and•half or heavy cream for a richer, creamier texture.
• Add a scoop of vanilla ice cream for an extra creamy treat.
• Blend in a banana for extra thickness and natural sweetness.
• Top with a dollop of whipped cream and a sprinkle of ground cinnamon.
• For an adult version, stir in a shot of rum or vodka.

The Orange Julius is a classic frothy, creamy, and sweet orange•flavored beverage. The combination of fresh orange juice, milk, and vanilla creates a refreshing and nostalgic treat. Adjust the ingredients to your taste preferences. Enjoy this delicious and easy•to•make drink!

115. Chai Latte:
Chai tea, milk, sugar, cinnamon, vanilla extract.

Ingredient:

- 2 cups milk (dairy, almond, oat, etc.)
- 2 chai tea bags or 2 tablespoons loose leaf chai tea
- 1•2 tablespoons granulated sugar (or to taste)
- 1/2 teaspoon ground cinnamon
- 1/4 teaspoon vanilla extract

Instructions:

1. In a small saucepan, heat the milk over medium heat until steaming and just beginning to simmer. Remove from heat.

2. Add the chai tea bags (or loose leaf tea) and let steep for 5•7 minutes, until the milk is infused with the chai flavor.

3. Remove the tea bags (or strain out the loose leaf tea) and return the chai•infused milk to the saucepan.

4. Whisk in the sugar, cinnamon, and vanilla extract until well combined and the sugar has dissolved.

5. If desired, use a milk frother or whisk vigorously to create a foamy texture.

6. Pour the chai latte into mugs.

7. Optionally, top with an extra sprinkle of cinnamon.

Variations:
- Use honey or maple syrup instead of granulated sugar.
- Add a pinch of ground cardamom or ginger for extra spice.
- Substitute half•and•half or heavy cream for a richer, creamier latte.
- Blend the chai latte with ice for a chilled, frappuccino•style drink.
- Top with whipped cream or a drizzle of caramel or chocolate sauce.

This homemade chai latte captures the warm, aromatic flavors of traditional chai tea. The combination of black tea, spices, and creamy milk creates a comforting and indulgent beverage. Adjust the sweetness to your taste preferences.

116. Pineapple Smoothie:
Pineapple, coconut milk, banana, ice, honey.

Ingredient:

- 1 cup fresh or frozen pineapple chunks
- 1 ripe banana
- 1 cup unsweetened coconut milk
- 1•2 tablespoons honey (or to taste)
- 1 cup ice cubes

Instructions:

1. In a blender, combine the pineapple chunks, banana, coconut milk, and honey.

2. Add the ice cubes and blend on high speed until smooth and creamy, about 1•2 minutes.

3. Taste and adjust sweetness as needed, adding more honey if desired.

4. Pour the pineapple smoothie into glasses and serve immediately.

Variations:
- Use plain Greek yogurt instead of coconut milk for a thicker, creamier texture.
- Add a handful of spinach or kale for extra nutrients.
- Substitute almond milk or oat milk for the coconut milk.
- Include a scoop of vanilla protein powder for a protein boost.
- Top with toasted coconut flakes, crushed pineapple, or a wedge of fresh pineapple.
- For a tropical twist, add a splash of rum or coconut rum.

This refreshing pineapple smoothie combines the sweet, tangy flavor of pineapple with the creaminess of coconut milk and the natural sweetness of banana. The honey adds an extra touch of sweetness. Enjoy this bright, tropical•inspired smoothie as a healthy breakfast or snack.

117. Strawberry Lemonade:
Strawberries, lemon juice, sugar, water, ice.

Ingredient:
- 1 lb fresh strawberries, hulled and sliced
- 1 cup freshly squeezed lemon juice (about 6•8 lemons)
- 1/2 cup granulated sugar
- 4 cups cold water
- Ice cubes

Instructions:

1. In a medium saucepan, combine the sliced strawberries and sugar. Mash the strawberries lightly with a potato masher or fork.

2. Place the saucepan over medium heat and cook, stirring occasionally, until the sugar has dissolved and the strawberries have released their juices, about 5•7 minutes.

3. Remove the saucepan from the heat and let the strawberry mixture cool completely.

4. Once cooled, strain the strawberry mixture through a fine•mesh sieve, pressing on the solids to extract as much juice as possible. Discard the solids.

5. In a large pitcher, combine the strained strawberry juice, lemon juice, and cold water. Stir until well mixed.

6. Taste and adjust sweetness as needed, adding more sugar if desired.

7. Fill glasses with ice cubes.

8. Pour the strawberry lemonade over the ice and serve immediately.

Variations:
- Use a combination of lemon and lime juice for a citrus twist.
- Add a few sprigs of fresh mint or basil for an herbal note.
- Blend the lemonade with ice for a slushy, frozen consistency.
- For an adult version, stir in a shot of vodka or gin.

The sweet•tart combination of fresh strawberries and lemon juice creates a refreshing and vibrant lemonade. Adjust the sugar to your taste preferences. Enjoy this homemade strawberry lemonade on a hot summer day!

Thank you for joining us on this culinary journey through ***"5-Ingredient Cookbook for College Students: Fast, Fresh, and Budget-Friendly Recipes for Students".*** We hope that this book has inspired you to step into the kitchen and discover the joys of cooking, even with a busy college schedule.

Key Takeaways

Throughout these pages, you've learned how simple and satisfying it can be to prepare meals using just five ingredients. You've explored a variety of dishes that are not only quick and easy but also nutritious and delicious. From breakfast boosters to sweet treats, you've now got a repertoire of recipes that fit perfectly into your hectic lifestyle.

Benefits Beyond the Kitchen

Cooking your own meals offers benefits that go beyond just eating well. It teaches you valuable skills like time management, budgeting, and creativity. It also provides a sense of accomplishment and independence, empowering you to take control of your health and wellbeing.

Continuing Your Culinary Adventure

As you move forward, remember that cooking is a skill that grows with practice. Don't be afraid to experiment with new ingredients or modify recipes to suit your taste. The five-ingredient philosophy is a great starting point, but feel free to expand your culinary horizons as you become more comfortable in the kitchen.

Staying Connected

We'd love to hear about your cooking experiences and see the delicious meals you've created. Connect with us on social media, share your favorite recipes, and join a community of fellow student chefs who are passionate about making great food with minimal fuss.

Thank you for choosing this cookbook as your culinary companion. We hope it has made your college cooking experience easier, more enjoyable, and incredibly tasty. Here's to many more delicious meals and happy memories in the kitchen!